TREATMENT MATCHING IN AL

Is alcoholism a treatable illness? Do different treatments work better for some alcoholics than for others? Is Alcoholics Anonymous the best road to recovery for alcoholics? Questions such as these formed the background to the research described in this ground-breaking book.

Project MATCH was a large-scale treatment evaluation study established by the US National Institute on Alcohol Abuse and Alcoholism to determine whether the treatment of alcoholism could be improved by matching different types of alcoholics with the most appropriate kinds of treatment. This book, edited by two of the principal investigators, is the first comprehensive report of Project MATCH, the largest treatment study ever conducted with alcoholics. It describes the rationale, methods, results, and implications of the study, and presents new findings about how treatment works, for whom it is most effective, and who does best in different kinds of treatment. It also offers some of the first scientific evidence of the effectiveness of Alcoholics Anonymous.

The audience for this book is broad, including researchers, clinicians, and policy makers in the field of alcoholism and addiction.

THOMAS F. BABOR is Professor and Chairman in the Department of Community Medicine and Health Care, University of Connecticut School of Medicine, where he was the scientific director of the Alcohol Research Center. He was principal investigator of the coordinating Center of Project MATCH, as well as of several other multicenter clinical trials of treatment for alcohol and drug abuse.

FRANCES K. DEL BOCA is Associate Professor in the Department of Psychology, and Director of Assessment at the Alcohol and Substance Use Research Institute, University of South Florida. She was co-principal investigator at the Coordinating Center for Project MATCH.

INTERNATIONAL RESEARCH MONOGRAPHS IN THE ADDICTIONS (IRMA)

Series Editor
Professor Griffith Edwards
National Addiction Centre
Institute of Psychiatry, London

A series of volumes presenting important research from major centers around the world on the basic sciences, both biological and behavioral, that have a bearing on the addictions, and also addressing the clinical and public health applications of such research. The series will cover alcohol, illicit drugs, psychotropics and tobacco, and is an important resource for clinicians, researchers and policy-makers.

Also in this series:

Cannabis and Cognitive Functioning
Nadia Solowij
ISBN 0 521 159114 7

Alcohol and the Community: A Systems Approach to Prevention
Harold D. Holder
ISBN 0 521 59187 2

A Community Reinforcement Approach to Addiction Treatment
Robert J. Meyers and William R. Miller
ISBN 0 521 77107 2

TREATMENT MATCHING IN ALCOHOLISM

Edited by

THOMAS F. BABOR
University of Connecticut School of Medicine

and

FRANCES K. DEL BOCA
University of South Florida

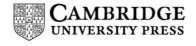
CAMBRIDGE
UNIVERSITY PRESS

CAMBRIDGE UNIVERSITY PRESS
Cambridge, New York, Melbourne, Madrid, Cape Town, Singapore,
São Paulo, Delhi, Dubai, Tokyo, Mexico City

Cambridge University Press
The Edinburgh Building, Cambridge CB2 8RU, UK

Published in the United States of America by Cambridge University Press, New York

www.cambridge.org
Information on this title: www.cambridge.org/9780521177269

First published 2003
First paperback edition 2010

A catalogue record for this publication is available from the British Library

Library of Congress Cataloguing in Publication Data

Treatment matching in alcoholism / edited by Thomas F. Babor and Frances K. Del Boca.
    p.   cm. – (International research monographs in the addictions)
Includes bibliographical references and index.
ISBN 0 521 65112 3
1. Alcoholism – Treatment.   I. Babor, Thomas.   II. Del Boca, Frances K.   III. Series.
RC565.T72 2002
616.861'06–dc21   2002067652

ISBN 978-0-521-65112-7 Hardback
ISBN 978-0-521-17726-9 Paperback

This book is dedicated to the people who made Project MATCH possible:

1726 research participants, 159 research personnel, 81 therapists, 14 therapy personnel, 8 collaborating investigators who were not members of the Project MATCH Research Group, 5 members of the Data Safety and Monitoring Board, 4 NIAAA support staff, 3 consultants, 2 editors' spouses

and Norma.

Contents

List of contributors   *page* ix
Note from Series Editor   xii
Preface   xiii

Part I Design and Implementation   1

1 Matching alcoholism treatment to client heterogeneity:
   the genesis of Project MATCH   3
   JOHN P. ALLEN, THOMAS F. BABOR, MARGARET E. MATTSON,
   AND RONALD M. KADDEN

2 Planning a multisite matching trial: organizational
   structure and research design   15
   FRANCES K. DEL BOCA, MARGARET E. MATTSON,
   RICHARD FULLER, AND THOMAS F. BABOR

3 Clinical assessment: measuring matching characteristics
   and treatment outcomes   29
   GERARD J. CONNORS, WILLIAM R. MILLER, RAYMOND F. ANTON,
   AND J. SCOTT TONIGAN

4 Therapies for matching: selection, development, implementation,
   and costs   42
   DENNIS M. DONOVAN, KATHLEEN M. CARROLL,
   RONALD M. KADDEN, CARLO C. DICLEMENTE,
   AND BRUCE J. ROUNSAVILLE

5 Client characteristics and implementation of the research
   protocol   62
   ALLEN ZWEBEN, FRANCES K. DEL BOCA, MARGARET E. MATTSON,
   AND BONNIE MCREE

6 The matching hypotheses: rationale and predictions   81
RONALD M. KADDEN, RICHARD LONGABAUGH,
AND PHILIP W. WIRTZ

Part II Findings   103

7 Primary treatment outcomes and matching effects:
Outpatient arm   105
ROBERT STOUT, FRANCES DEL K. BOCA, JOSEPH CARBONARI,
ROBERT RYCHTARIK, MARK D. LITT, AND NED L. COONEY

8 Primary treatment outcomes and matching effects:
Aftercare arm   135
CARRIE L. RANDALL, FRANCES K. DEL BOCA,
MARGARET E. MATTSON, ROBERT RYCHTARIK, NED L. COONEY,
DENNIS M. DONOVAN, RICHARD LONGABAUGH,
AND PHILIP W. WIRTZ

9 Treatment effects across multiple dimensions of outcome   150
THOMAS F. BABOR, KAREN STEINBERG, ALLEN ZWEBEN,
RON CISLER, ROBERT STOUT, J. SCOTT TONIGAN,
RAYMOND F. ANTON, AND JOHN P. ALLEN

10 A look inside treatment: therapist effects, the therapeutic
alliance, and the process of intentional behavior change   166
CARLO C. DICLEMENTE, KATHLEEN M. CARROLL,
WILLIAM R. MILLER, GERARD J. CONNORS,
AND DENNIS M. DONOVAN

11 Participation and involvement in Alcoholics Anonymous   184
J. SCOTT TONIGAN, GERARD J. CONNORS,
AND WILLIAM R. MILLER

Part III Conclusions and Implications   205

12 Summary and conclusions   207
WILLIAM R. MILLER AND RICHARD LONGABAUGH

13 Clinical and scientific implications of Project MATCH   222
NED L. COONEY, THOMAS F. BABOR, CARLO C. DICLEMENTE,
AND FRANCES K. DEL BOCA

Appendix Personnel and facilities affiliated with Project MATCH   238

References   245
Index   265

Contributors

John P. Allen
NIAAA, 6000 Executive Blvd,
Willco Building, Suite 505,
Rockville, MD 20892-7003,
USA

Raymond F. Anton
Center for Drug and Alcohol
Programs (CDAP),
Medical University of South Carolina,
171 Ashley Avenue,
Charleston, SC 29425-0742,
USA

Thomas F. Babor
University of Connecticut Health
Center,
Department of Community Medicine
and Health Care,
263 Farmington Avenue,
Farmington, CT 06030-6325,
USA

Joseph Carbonari
University of Houston,
Department of Psychology,
4800 Calhoun,
Houston, TX 77204-5341,
USA

Kathleen M. Carroll
Yale University,
Department of Psychiatry,
VA CT Healthcare Cnt (151D),
950 Campbell Avenue,
West Haven, CT 06516,
USA

Ron Cisler
Center for Addiction and Behavioral
Health Research,
University of Wisconsin–Milwaukee
School of Social Welfare,
2400 E. Hartford Avenue,
1147 Enderis Hall,
Milwaukee, WI 53201,
USA

Ned L. Cooney
VA Connecticut Healthcare System
(116A-3),
555 Willard Avenue,
Newington, CT 06111,
USA

Gerard J. Connors
Research Institute on Addictions,
1021 Main Street,
Buffalo, NY 14203,
USA

Frances K. Del Boca
University of South Florida,
Department of Psychology PCD
4118G,
4200 E. Fowler Avenue,
Tampa, FL 32620-8200,
USA

Carlo C. DiClemente
University of Maryland,
Baltimore County,
Department of Psychology,
1000 Hilltop Circle,
Baltimore, MD 21250,
USA

Dennis M. Donovan
Alcohol and Drug Abuse Institute,
University of Washington,
3937 15th Avenue, NE,
Seattle, WA 98105-6696,
USA

Richard Fuller
NIAAA, 6000 Executive Blvd,
Willco Building, Suite 505,
Rockville, MD 20892-7003,
USA

Ronald M. Kadden
University of Connecticut Health
Center,
Department of Psychiatry,
263 Farmington Avenue,
Farmington, CT 06030-2103,
USA

Mark D. Litt
University of Connecticut Health
Center,
Department of Behavioral Sciences,
263 Farmington Avenue,
Farmington, CT 06030-3910,
USA

Richard Longabaugh
Brown University, Potter Building,
Center for Alcohol and Addiction
Studies,
345 Blackstone Blvd,
Box G-BH – Rm 303,
Providence, RI 02912,
USA

Margaret E. Mattson
NIAAA, 6000 Executive Blvd,
Willco Building, Suite 505,
Rockville, MD 20892-7003,
USA

Bonnie McRee
University of Connecticut Health
Center,
Department of Community Medicine
and Health Care,
263 Farmington Avenue,
Farmington, CT 06030-6325,
USA

William R. Miller
University of New Mexico,
Department of Psychology,
Logan Hall, Terrace and Redondo,
Albuquerque, NM 87131-1161,
USA

Carrie L. Randall
Center for Drug and Alcohol
Programs (CDAP),
Medical University of South Carolina,
171 Ashley Avenue,
Charleston, SC 29425-0742,
USA

Bruce J. Rounsaville
Yale University,
Department of Psychiatry,
VA CT Healthcare Cnt (151D),
950 Campbell Avenue,
West Haven, CT 06516,
USA

Robert Rychtarik
Research Institute on Addictions,
1021 Main Street,
Buffalo, NY 14203,
USA

Karen Steinberg
University of Connecticut Health
Center,
Department of Psychiatry,
263 Farmington Avenue,
Farmington, CT 06030-1410,
USA

Robert Stout
Decision Sciences Institute,
120 Wayland Avenue,
Suite 7,
Providence, RI 02906,
USA

J. Scott Tonigan
University of New Mexico,
Center on Alcoholism,
Substance Abuse and Addictions,
2350 Alamo SE,
Albuquerque, NM 87106,
USA

Philip W. Wirtz
George Washington University,
James Monroe Hall,
Room 203,
Department of Management Science,
2115 G. Street, NW,
Washington, DC 20052,
USA

Allen Zweben
Center for Addiction and Behavioral
Health Research,
University of Wisconsin–Milwaukee
School of Social Welfare,
2400 E. Hartford Avenue,
1147 Enderis Hall,
Milwaukee, WI 53201,
USA

Note from Series Editor

The International Research Monographs in the Addictions (IRMA) was set up by Cambridge University Press with a closely defined intention. We aim to offer authors the opportunity for book-length statements on their work and methodologies, an invitation to develop ideas in greater detail than can ever be done in any sequence of separate papers, the chance to act as their own critics, and an invitation to scan the horizons. To readers of this series we want to offer scholarly material of a high standard which is strictly refereed and well presented. IRMA asks its authors to address the policy and treatment worlds. We fuss about these monographs being readable and hope that they are good to hold in the hand. I believe that Thomas Babor, Frances Del Boca and their colleagues have produced a text which absolutely fulfils the founding intentions.

MATCH is near-contemporary research although it already has about it the glow of a classic, and a place booked in history. As Babor and Del Boca say in their preface, a book like this can compel its own logic in the process of its writing – 'the reader for the first time will be able to grasp not only what we learned about treatment matching, but also what we learned about the limits of clinical science.' That kind of writing is a wonderfully creative act, an affirmation of scientific integrity, and constitutes a true service to the field.

GRIFFITH EDWARDS

Preface

Some of the most contentious ideological debates in the history of addiction science were conducted during the 1960s and 1970s over clinical questions like the following. Is alcoholism a disease? Can a person, once becoming an alcoholic, ever drink moderately again? Is Alcoholics Anonymous the best road to recovery for all alcoholics? No clinical study of therapeutic interventions could escape the sensitivities and sensibilities of the different constituency groups that became part of the burgeoning field of addiction treatment. Many academics were skeptical about the conventional wisdom of the disease concept of alcoholism, and recovering persons learned to distrust academics who presented evidence that problem drinkers could learn to drink moderately.

In many respects, Project MATCH is a product of these divergent views of the reality that is alcoholism treatment. But, by the 1990s, when the Project MATCH Research Group was formed, American academics were recognizing the need to formulate more precise research questions and to test them with the new clinical trial methodologies that were contributing so much to the advancement of clinical practice in medicine and psychiatry. In this case, the research question concerned whether treatment effectiveness could be improved substantially by matching different types of alcoholics with the most appropriate kinds of treatment. The Project MATCH Research Group was assembled by the US National Institute on Alcohol Abuse and Alcoholism (NIAAA) in the hope that a large-scale treatment evaluation study would accomplish for the field of alcoholism research what clinical epidemiology had done for medicine. The participating investigators were selected on the strength of their grant proposals. Each proposal described the investigator's approach to treatment matching research, as well as his or her past accomplishments in this area.

However, unlike the funding of smaller and less ambitious research grants, the monies provided for Project MATCH did not require the investigators to specify in advance a final research plan to study treatment matching. It was assumed that once the investigators and their research teams were selected, the process of defining the research questions and designing the study would be entrusted to the group, rather than to a few expert consultants or to the institute staff themselves.

As the process unfolded, it became clear that the Project MATCH Research Group would not always speak with one voice. The differences among the investigators were often dramatic, and most had a specific bias about how to study matching and which questions to investigate. Indeed, when the group was first assembled, they resembled the Seven Blind Men of Hindustan, each speaking with conviction about the matching phenomena they had discovered through their own limited explorations.

What is remarkable about the process of this investigation is the extent to which the desire to find the right answer, rather than the need to prove that one idea was superior to another, eventually emerged as the *raison d'être* for Project MATCH. If skepticism is the hallmark of good science, then it is what both attracted the investigators to the project and kept them honest in its implementation. To come to grips with matching theory, it was necessary to grapple with scientific methodology, establish rigorous rules of evidence, and take into consideration the plight of the millions of people whose lives are ruined by alcohol misuse. All of this entered into the intellectual process of planning, executing, and interpreting the results of the study. If it matters whether there is such a thing as truth, whether honest inquiry is possible, and whether there is a real difference between knowledge and ideology, then we feel that Project MATCH has succeeded admirably, both in style and in substance.

In editing this book, we have done our best to avoid academic jargon and unnecessary technical language. We have tried to speak to clinicians as well as research scientists by bringing together the full range of findings that have emerged out of a decade of work on the project. The findings of Project MATCH were released sequentially in over a hundred scientific publications and presentations; initial impressions of the study were often based on small parts of the project instead of on the total picture. Unlike the first outcome paper that was published in 1997 (Project MATCH Research Group, 1997a), the cumulative corpus of findings tells a far more complex story about alcoholism treatment and how it works. We feel that only after all the articles have been published is it possible to gain a broader perspective on what we found and what it means. To that end, we have assembled within this volume a complete description of the origins of the trial as well as its design, implementation, and results. Part I describes the background to the study, giving particular attention to the technology for evaluating different kinds of psychotherapy and the types of clients most likely to respond to them. Part II presents the findings, some of which are being reported for the first time (see especially Chapters 9, 10, and 11). Finally, Part III describes the study's conclusions and implications.

How we got to this point is told only in part in the pages of this book. It was in 1998 that an epiphany of sorts occurred when representatives of the Project MATCH Research Group were asked to present a comprehensive summary of the findings at a 2-day symposium in Leeds, England (Ashton, 1999). Instead of the 1-hour or 2-hour format that we had been accustomed to use in the past, the Leeds conference allowed the investigators to tell their story in numbers, words, anecdotes, and intuitions, and it permitted the audience of clinicians and researchers to 'Meet the Matchmakers' on their own terms. The results of that meeting convinced us that the best format for describing what we did and what we found was not the narrowly focused journal article, but rather the compelling logic of a book like this one. By weaving together disparate findings from all facets of this ambitious project, we believe that the reader for the first time will be able to grasp not only what we learned about treatment matching, but also what we learned about the limits of clinical science. Despite the international interest in Project MATCH, a key feature of its design and execution is that it came out of a scientific and clinical context that was distinctly American. How this context influenced the study's research questions, experimental methods, and scientific conclusions is an intriguing question that is taken up at the end of this book.

We would be remiss if we did not attempt at least a partial acknowledgment of the many people who contributed to Project MATCH over a 10-year period. NIAAA deserves credit for its decision to move alcoholism treatment research into the realm of multisite clinical trials. We are especially indebted to Dr Enoch Gordis, Director of NIAAA, for his support of Project MATCH, and to Dr Richard K. Fuller of NIAAA for his invaluable guidance over the course of the project. The contributions of the individual investigators who comprise the Project MATCH Research Group cannot be overstated; each chapter in this volume represents the collective efforts of this entire group. The credit for an endeavor of this magnitude must also be shared with the very large number of co-investigators, statistical consultants, project coordinators, research assistants, therapists, and collaborating treatment facilities who bore the day-to-day responsibility of making the project work. Finally, we acknowledge the thoughtful oversight provided by the project's Data Monitoring Board, and the editorial work done by Norma Carbonari for the Publication Committee. The names of all those who contributed to Project MATCH in these capacities appear in the appendix to this book.

On a more personal level, we would like to acknowledge the efforts of a handful of individuals who contributed to the preparation of this volume. These include Deborah Talamini, who, with the assistance of Katherine Hedgspeth and Dominique Morisano, managed the production of the book; Dr Robert Stout, who prepared the figures depicting the study's primary results; and the core research staff of the Coordinating Center, Bonnie McRee, Cynthia Mohr, and Janice Vendetti. We also appreciate the guidance and wisdom of Griffith Edwards.

On behalf of the Project MATCH Research Group, we hope that this book will serve as a tribute to the pursuit of scientific knowledge about the nature and treatment of alcoholism.

THOMAS F. BABOR
FRANCES K. DEL BOCA

Part I

Design and Implementation

1

Matching alcoholism treatment to client heterogeneity: the genesis of Project MATCH

JOHN P. ALLEN, THOMAS F. BABOR, MARGARET E. MATTSON,
AND RONALD M. KADDEN

Clinical trials are a special form of scientific research designed to test causal hypotheses about the efficacy of a particular treatment for a specific condition. By the late 1980s, clinical trials of alcoholism treatment had advanced to the point where new hypotheses had arisen about the efficacy of matching specific treatments to particular types of alcoholics. This chapter describes the origins of the matching hypothesis in alcoholism treatment research and the genesis of Project MATCH, one of the largest clinical trials of alcoholism treatment ever undertaken. It reviews definitions and forms of matching as well as previous matching studies.

The idea of matching highly specific therapeutic interventions to the unique characteristics of each alcoholic is not a recent phenomenon. In the late nineteenth century the practice of homeopathic medicine was applied to alcoholism according to the principle of *similia similibus curantur*, or patients are best treated with agents that are similar to their symptoms. Using a crude typology of alcoholism that has some resemblance to contemporary classification theories, Dr Gallavardin, a French physician, argued that there are two kinds of 'drunkenness,' which require quite different treatments. The first, acquired drunkenness, was considered the easier to cure by means of a few 'remedies' clearly indicated in each individual. In order to cure the second form of alcoholism, hereditary drunkenness, the author suggested preventive interventions '. . . before the tendency to drunkenness has manifested itself,' by administering, for several years, no fewer than 13 remedies, including arsenic, opium, and petroleum (Gallavardin, 1890, pp. 44–5). In addition to the careful dosing of pharmacological agents, the physician was cautioned to use a motivational approach that begins with the following advice: 'No reproaches should be addressed to the person under treatment, even though he might

3

deserve them richly, and in conversation no allusion should be made to his vices or failings' (Gallavardin, 1890, p. 71). For more than 150 years, alcoholism has been treated by a wide variety of pharmacological and psychological interventions (White, 1998), many of which have been designed, like Dr Gallavardin's homeopathic remedies, for specific types of alcoholics. However, it was not until the 1980s that the matching hypothesis was formulated with sufficient conceptual rigor to permit a scientific test of its validity. This chapter describes the genesis of the matching hypothesis and of Project MATCH, the most ambitious attempt to date to test its scientific validity and clinical relevance.

For most of the twentieth century, the matching of therapeutic interventions to the needs of the patient was impeded by the lack of a commonly accepted way to classify alcoholics into distinct groups, and by the lack of a systematic theory that would suggest how types of alcoholics could be matched to the most appropriate treatment (Babor & Lauerman, 1986). By the late 1970s, there was a general impression in the public mind, as well as in professional circles in the USA, that alcoholism was a treatable disease, in part because of the optimistic message of Alcoholics Anonymous, and in part because of the rapid expansion of professional treatment programs. A strong constituency was formed around the loosely assembled system of treatment programs that had emerged through the rapid increase in public and private reimbursement for alcoholism treatment. That constituency tended to interpret the growing research literature as favorable to the idea that treatment is effective, whereas a small number of critics expressed doubts about treatment in general, and about the limited support for specific treatment interventions in particular (Emrick & Hansen, 1983; Miller & Hester, 1986a). Out of this debate emerged a third perspective, that of treatment matching. This view is summarized most clearly in the US Institute of Medicine's 1990 report on alcoholism treatment:

There is no single treatment approach that is effective for all persons with alcohol problems. A number of treatment methods show promise in particular groups. Reason for optimism in the treatment of alcohol problems lies in the range of promising alternatives that are available, *each of which may be optimal for different types of individuals* (Institute of Medicine, 1990, p. 147).

During the 1970s and 1980s, accumulating evidence raised the possibility of significantly improving treatment outcomes by assigning alcoholics to types and levels of care specific to their needs and characteristics (Mattson & Allen, 1991; Mattson et al., 1994; Allen & Kadden, 1995). Although a number of alcoholism treatment approaches had shown benefit, no specific type of intervention had been demonstrated to be consistently and definitively superior (Hester & Miller, 1989).

Miller (1989b) speculated that, in at least some instances, treatment failure might indicate that the right treatment approach was not utilized and that client–treatment matching would perhaps both avoid unnecessary therapeutic failures and increase cost-effectiveness. Under such a scenario, rather than competing with one another for *all* alcoholic clients, treatment programs and therapists would instead seek the type of clients for whom their approach was most effective. Without doubt, implementation of this advice would require a substantial knowledge base regarding client attributes that influence treatment effectiveness. In addition, various aspects of treatment such as modality, intensity, duration, format, setting, goal, and therapist characteristics would have to be considered in making decisions about treatment matching (Miller & Cooney, 1994). Finally, a systematic strategy for matching individuals to available treatments would need to be developed.

The genesis of Project MATCH can only be understood in the context of these issues. To describe the rationale behind the initiation of Project MATCH, it is first necessary to discuss recent developments in definitions of matching, matching strategies, stages of matching, and predictors of treatment outcome.

Definitions and forms of matching

Alcoholism is a term with many definitions and even more meanings (Jellinek, 1960). It generally refers to a chronic condition characterized by impaired control over drinking, increased tolerance to the effects of alcohol, a physical withdrawal state (when alcohol consumption is stopped or reduced), and a learned preference for alcohol over almost every other rewarding activity in a person's life. The term alcoholism is used synonymously in this book with the more formal psychiatric disorder, called the alcohol dependence syndrome (American Psychiatric Association, 1987). Despite the common clinical features shared by persons who have developed alcohol dependence, alcoholics differ among themselves in many ways. Some of these differences have little to do with alcohol: age, motivation, spirituality, personality, and cognitive style. Other differences distinguish alcoholics in terms of alcohol-related features, such as severity of alcohol involvement and early versus late onset of alcohol dependence. It is this heterogeneity among alcoholics that makes treatment matching a particularly exciting approach to the development of more effective clinical services. The matching hypothesis predicts that alcoholics who are appropriately matched to treatments will show better outcomes than those who are unmatched or mismatched (Glaser, 1980; Finney & Moos, 1986; Lindström, 1992). As discussed in more detail in Chapter 6, a number of specific matching effects can be predicted on the basis of what has been found in previous research on alcoholics (Longabaugh et al., 1994b).

According to Glaser and Skinner (1981), matching is above all a practical approach, defined as '. . . the deliberate and consistent attempt to select a specific candidate for a specific method of intervention in order to achieve specific goals' (p. 302). This definition implies that matching requires the specification of different types of clients who are most appropriate for different types of treatment in order to achieve different kinds of treatment goals.

A distinction should be made between *predictors* of positive outcome regardless of the type of treatment employed, and *client matching factors* that exert differential effects depending on the type of treatment delivered. Figure 1.1 displays three types of results that may arise from a study contrasting two treatments, one 'gender focused' (i.e., designed to meet the special needs of women) and one 'generic' (i.e., designed to apply to both men and women equally well).

The upper panel in Figure 1.1 shows the effect of an outcome predictor (gender) which does not produce a matching effect. The outcomes are better for females regardless of the therapy they receive. The middle panel illustrates one way that ordinal matching may occur. An ordinal interaction is indicated when nonparallel regression lines do not intersect within the research range of interest. Here, females benefit more from gender-specific treatment than from the generic therapy, whereas males experience approximately equal levels of success in both types of treatment.

Disordinal matching is observed when the treatment outcomes reverse between clients having low levels versus high levels of the characteristic under study (lower panel of Fig. 1.1). In the illustration, gender-focused treatment is beneficial for females but not for males, whereas generic treatment is more beneficial for males than for females.

In general, disordinal matching effects are the most interesting from both theoretical and practical perspectives. The discovery of disordinal matching effects between distinct treatments and different types or levels of client characteristics is considered strong evidence for a theory of differential treatment response. Moreover, such findings could have tremendous

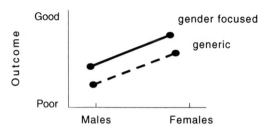

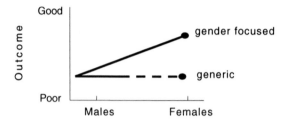

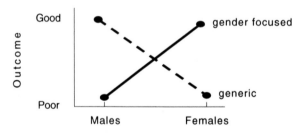

Figure 1.1 Illustration of hypothetical matching effects of gender-focused versus generic treatment with male and female alcoholic clients (adapted from Longabaugh et al., 1994b).

practical significance, suggesting which clients to assign to the specific treatment modalities for maximum benefit.

Matching strategies

For years, practicing clinicians in alcoholism treatment have engaged in several forms of client–treatment matching. Clients are often triaged to different settings, durations, and intensities of care, for example according to their need for detoxification, the severity of dependence on other drugs in addition to alcohol, and diagnoses of concurrent anxiety, depression, or other psychiatric disorders. In some instances, the problems are severe and therefore the clinical decisions are obvious. However, in the case of less severe or more subtle problems, treatment decisions are more difficult and, in current practice, depend largely on the clinical judgment and theoretical perspective of the decision maker. Lindström (1992) has recommended that treatment selection be based both on practitioners' clinical assessments and on data from standardized diagnostic instruments. Based on clinical practice and theoretical considerations, at least six strategies have been suggested in the investigation of client–treatment matching (Institute of Medicine, 1989).

1. *Reliance on clinical judgment.* Clinical judgment is perhaps the most typical strategy for treatment matching, although it has received virtually no research attention. Clients are typically referred to treatment by doctors, social service agencies or, more recently in the USA, by managed care programs. Some individuals are presented with a limited range of options because of treatment mandates from the legal system. Because the referral process is often arbitrary, and little is known about clinician decision making when it enters into this process, systematic research on this strategy could have practical value.

2. *Self-selection or the 'cafeteria' approach.* This strategy, first proposed by Ewing (1977), relies on the client to select the most appropriate treatment from a range of options. It is assumed that clients will select the form of treatment that is most compatible with their medical needs, personal preferences, and financial resources. With the development of assessment centers charged with the use of standard patient placement criteria, the cafeteria approach could be contrasted with other referral methods to determine whether self-matching provides better outcomes and greater satisfaction with treatment.

3. *Matching guided by exploratory data analysis.* In this type of 'feedback design' (Institute of Medicine, 1989), treatment assignment procedures are studied within an existing network of programs to identify the assumptions behind the matching strategies that are employed and their impact on outcomes. After evaluating the relative outcomes with matched and unmatched or mismatched clients, changes are made to

improve the treatment system. The effects of these changes on outcomes can then be evaluated.

4. *Matching guided by theoretically derived hypotheses.* This strategy relies on the cumulative evidence of research to suggest the kinds of treatments most likely to produce favorable outcomes with different types of clients. An example is the assignment of clients with antisocial personality disorder to cognitive–behavioral treatment, based on the assumption (e.g., Kadden et al., 1989) that these patients have a need for consistency and structure and therefore will have better outcomes with this kind of therapy. This is the approach ultimately chosen by Project MATCH, in part because it showed promise to advance basic knowledge about treatment, and in part because it lends itself to rigorous methodological evaluation.

5. *Matching according to professional guidelines.* In response to concerns about the inappropriate use of expensive residential treatment, 'patient placement criteria' have been developed for adults (Gartner & Mee-Lee, 1995) and adolescents (Babor et al., 1991) to standardize the way in which clients are assigned to different types and intensities of care. For example, criteria proposed by the American Society of Addiction Medicine (1991) specify the conditions under which clients should be matched to outpatient, intensive outpatient, partial hospital, and inpatient treatment. The decision to refer the client to a particular level of care is based on such considerations as acute intoxication, withdrawal symptoms, medical conditions, psychiatric problems, acceptance of treatment, relapse potential, and recovery environment. This kind of matching strategy is primarily a practical guide to the choice of an appropriate treatment setting. Because settings differ in the quality and content of the treatment they deliver, the study of matching to levels of care and treatment settings is unlikely to produce useful information about the efficacy or the underlying processes of treatment matching.

6. *Stepped-care approaches.* Another approach to matching is based on the notion that clients should initially be assigned to the least intensive level of care that is appropriate, and then 'stepped up' to more intensive treatment settings if they do not respond (Institute of Medicine, 1990). In this way, information regarding the most appropriate matches for various types of clients is developed empirically, based on accumulating clinical experience. To date, this approach has not been thoroughly evaluated.

Although each of these approaches is worthy of investigation, previous research has suggested that hypothesis-driven studies using controlled experimental designs are not only the most appropriate initial approach for the identification of matching effects, but also the best way to identify causal mechanisms (Skinner, 1981).

Stages of matching

Ideally, the process of matching should involve comprehensive assessment, negotiation of treatment goals, selection of an appropriate level of treatment, choice of an intervention, arrangements for the maintenance of treatment gains, and follow-up assessment.

An Institute of Medicine committee (1989) identified four areas that represent these different stages in the continuum of care. These stages are important to consider in any attempt to evaluate the efficacy of client–treatment matching.

1. *Matching before treatment starts.* As noted above, the selection of treatment for a particular client may occur in a variety of ways. Although little research has been conducted on this topic, it is likely that program marketing, informal referral networks, and geographic proximity are important determinants. More recently, matching to providers and settings has increasingly been brought under the control of managed care companies. A considerable degree of matching seems to occur before treatment is initiated as a result of program specialization, i.e., the tailoring of programs to suit the assumed needs of such population groups as adolescents, women, war veterans, gay men and lesbians, the homeless and people arrested for driving under the influence of alcohol.

2. *Matching at the initiation of treatment.* As suggested by the American Society of Addiction Medicine Patient Placement Criteria (American Society of Addiction Medicine, 1991), there are a number of different levels and intensities of care to which clients could be matched, based on their needs and characteristics at the initiation of treatment. Ranging from brief interventions to medically managed intensive inpatient care, matching at this stage is usually related to the intensity of care and is closely linked to specific settings, such as outpatient clinics and residential rehabilitation centers.

3. *Matching during the treatment process.* Although many programs claim

to deliver specific kinds of treatment, most residential and outpatient programs in the USA seem to offer a standard mix of group therapy, individual counseling, patient education, and attendance at AA meetings. Although the Twelve Step approach has had a major influence on the overall philosophy of many programs, most controlled clinical studies have been conducted on matching to specific treatment modalities, such as cognitive–behavioral relapse prevention therapy and interactive group therapy.

4. *Matching following the rehabilitation intervention.* The post-treatment environment has been identified as an important factor in treatment outcome (McLachlan, 1974), and evidence suggests that different types of clients respond differently to the type of aftercare they receive (Finney et al., 1980; Kadden et al., 1989).

If the randomized clinical trial is considered the best way to establish matching relationships and to discover the mechanisms underlying treatment, then the stage at which matching is evaluated needs to be chosen carefully. To maximize the amount of experimental control and to minimize extraneous factors that could influence outcomes independent of matching, the Project MATCH investigators concluded that matching during and after treatment would be the most fruitful stages to study.

Previous treatment matching studies

The matching concept has been applied to many areas of intervention, such as medicine, psychotherapy, and education, with varying degrees of success. A report from the Collaborative Research Program on the Treatment of Depression identified several client characteristics that predict differential success with either psychotherapy or pharmacotherapy (Sotsky et al., 1991), thus supporting the concept of matching. Early work in educational applications gave rise to the phrase 'aptitude–treatment interaction' (ATI), a term now widely used in the psychotherapy literature, although it is not common parlance in the alcoholism field (Dance & Neufeld, 1988). An exhaustive review of ATI research in psychotherapy settings noted some support for matching, especially in the treatment of anxiety disorders and depression (Dance & Neufeld, 1988). Nevertheless, clinical research on ATIs has yet to provide a well-documented basis for differential treatment selection (Beutler, 1991).

Although many alcohol studies have produced findings relevant to matching, few have been designed explicitly to test matching hypotheses. Early efforts directed at treatment matching focused on the identification of predictors of favorable treatment outcomes, based on the limited number of measures available at the time clients were admitted to treatment. As the amount of alcoholism treatment research has grown over the years, investigators have benefited from the increasing sophistication of research designs, statistical analysis techniques, outcome measures, assessment techniques, treatment interventions, and matching hypotheses.

A 1994 review article (Mattson et al., 1994) identified 31 studies that provided empirical support for client–treatment matching with alcoholism treatment. There was, however, considerable variation in the treatments employed in this research. Only three therapy types were studied often enough to suggest matching effects with some degree of confidence: (1) cognitive–behavioral approaches, (2) interpersonal or relationally oriented modalities, and (3) treatments characterized by higher levels of intensity.

Various combinations of cognitive–behavioral/coping skills approaches have been studied in matching research. Highly structured coping skills training, as described in the manual-driven approach of Monti et al. (1989), appears more beneficial for high-severity (Type B) alcoholics (Litt et al., 1992) and for those with greater degrees of psychiatric severity and sociopathy (Kadden et al., 1989; Cooney et al., 1991). Focused training to cope with high-risk drinking situations seems more helpful for those clients who can identify specific types of high-risk situations, compared to those whose drinking appears less under stimulus control (Annis & Davis, 1989). Communication skills training has been found to be more effective for clients who are less educated, have stronger urges to drink, and have high levels of anxiety, and high-anxiety participants fared worse if given mood management rather than communication skills training (Rohsenow et al., 1991).

With respect to relationally focused interventions, therapy designed to improve interpersonal interactions seems more effective with low-severity (Type A) alcoholics (Litt et al., 1992), as well as with clients who have low levels of anxiety, lower urges to drink, good role-playing skills (Kadden et al., 1992b), less sociopathy, and greater psychiatric severity (Kadden et al., 1989; Cooney et al., 1991). Likewise, Longabaugh et al. (1994a) found that clients diagnosed as having antisocial personality disorder did less well in relationship enhancement therapy than in extended cognitive therapy. Conjoint couples therapy utilizing coping skills training was more beneficial for those who scored higher on a personality measure of autonomy (McKay et al., 1993).

Intensity reflects a dimension of treatment that is often associated with the frequency, duration, or setting of the intervention. Clients found to benefit from more intense interventions have been variously described as socially unstable (Welte et al., 1981), socially unstable but intellectually intact (Kissen et al., 1970), high in psychiatric severity or social instability (Pettinati et al., 1993), gamma-type alcoholics (Orford et al., 1976), externally controlled (Hartman et al., 1988), and behaviorally impaired due to drinking (Lyons et al., 1982). While clearly tenable, the belief that greater severity of problems justifies more intense treatment remains tentative because most of the studies on which this assumption is based have confounded intensity of treatment with type of intervention.

Considerable attention has been focused on the adequacy of research methodology in studying matching (Mattson et al., 1994). Indeed, many of the earlier studies, although provocative, were not sufficiently robust to warrant clinical application and suffered from various methodological shortcomings. One of the most common limitations has been insufficient measurement of the underlying mechanisms hypothesized to account for anticipated client–treatment interactions. Also lacking has been an internal theory or framework to judge the plausibility of the observed matching (or mismatching) effect. Other methodological issues include statistical power, strategies for data analysis, factors related to selection of client, treatment, and outcome variables, integrity and intensity of the treatments, and the range of variability for each of the characteristics studied (Smith & Sechrest, 1991; Snow, 1991).

Rationale for Project MATCH

In response to expert reports and keen interest from the scientific community, treatment providers, and legislators, the US National Institute on Alcohol Abuse and Alcoholism (NIAAA), after extensive deliberation, determined in 1988 that the potential benefit of client–treatment matching was sufficient to initiate a rigorous, large-scale, randomized trial to assess its overall value as a treatment strategy and to quantify the effects of specific types of matches. A concept paper outlining research goals and project management requirements was prepared by NIAAA staff and unanimously approved by a peer review group. The cooperative agreement mechanism was chosen to support the trial. In contrast to more traditional investigator-initiated funding arrangements, the cooperative agreement facilitates collaboration between institute staff and researchers, and is conducive to the close cross-site coordination needed in a multisite clinical trial. A Request for Applications was issued in 1989 and nine clinical research units and a coordinating center were funded. Begun in 1989 and concluded in 1998, Project MATCH (Matching Alcoholism Treatments to Client Heterogeneity) was designed to determine if varying types of alcohol-dependent clients respond differentially to alternative interventions. The remaining chapters in this book elaborate upon the research design, its implementation, the findings, and their implications.

2

Planning a multisite matching trial: organizational structure and research design

FRANCES K. DEL BOCA, MARGARET E. MATTSON, RICHARD
FULLER, AND THOMAS F. BABOR

The planning of a multisite clinical trial of treatment matching requires
organized procedures to guide decision making about the research goals and
the experimental design of the study. This chapter describes the organizational
structure of Project MATCH, the research design, and the rationales behind
the choices that were made. Operating within the framework of a cooperative
agreement among 23 investigators, agency staff and consultants, the Project
MATCH Research Group developed a research design consisting of two
parallel matching studies (Outpatient and Aftercare) that differed in terms of
their recruitment methods and the treatment stage of study participants. Three
theoretically derived psychosocial interventions, Cognitive–Behavioral
Therapy, Motivational Enhancement Therapy, and Twelve Step Facilitation,
were selected for use in a randomized clinical trial of client–treatment
matching. Follow-up evaluations were conducted every 3 months during the
first year after treatment, and again 3 years after treatment in the Outpatient
sample. The chapter closes with a view of Project MATCH as a cooperative
agreement among investigators to pursue the meaning of the matching
hypothesis.

Although multisite, randomized clinical trials have become standard practice within the US National Institutes of Health, the National Institute on
Alcohol Abuse and Alcoholism (NIAAA) had little experience with this
type of clinical research at the time Project MATCH was initiated. Project
MATCH afforded an opportunity to establish a model for developing a
methodology and an administrative framework for conducting clinical
trials within the institute. Such a model would have to address a variety of
issues involving organizational structure, decision making, cross-site communication, and coordination. In the absence of a clear blueprint, work-
able structures and processes evolved as collaborating investigators confronted the many decisions entailed in developing a common research

design and in implementing a multisite project. The purpose of this chapter is to describe the organizational structure of the trial and to provide an overview of the Project MATCH research design.

Rationale for a multisite clinical trial

The basic framework for Project MATCH was sketched in the original concept paper prepared by NIAAA staff. The project was structured as a multisite clinical trial that would address the limitations of prior treatment matching research that are identified in Chapter 1. Multisite clinical trials offer several advantages over single-site studies. First, they allow rapid recruitment of large participant samples that are more heterogeneous than those typically used in single-site studies. Rapid recruitment decreases the risk that the subject pool will change during the course of the trial. Sample heterogeneity increases the chances that research findings will generalize to new populations. In a study of treatment matching, client diversity is also important because it assures adequate variation on characteristics that are expected to be differentially related to treatment outcomes.

Second, the larger sample size of a multisite clinical trial increases statistical power, thereby enhancing the possibility that client–treatment interactions will be found. Over the past decade, research into behavioral and medical interventions has often been criticized for insufficient power due to inadequate sample sizes (Cohen, 1988; Kazdin & Bass, 1989; Lipsey, 1990).

A third advantage of multisite trials over single-site investigations is the wealth of clinical, statistical, and methodological expertise brought to the task by the collaborating investigators, each of whom is likely to contribute unique skills, knowledge, and creative ideas.

While offering important advantages, multisite trials entail significant challenges as well. These include the need to control costs, maintain fidelity to the treatment protocol across dispersed settings, coordinate staff training and data collection, and assure the cooperation of a large number of researchers, none of whom 'owns' the trial. In the process of developing a consensus about the research design, the number of research questions that could be addressed in a series of smaller studies is reduced. As a consequence, decision making involves setting priorities and making hard choices regarding the investment of research capital. The start-up time for multisite trials is likely to be longer, requiring coordination of a large number of Institutional Review Boards or other panels dealing with human subjects' issues. Finally, the resolution of problems within the context of a group process, rather than by a few individuals, is likely to take longer, although decisions may be more carefully considered (see Fuller et al., 1994, for a more complete discussion of the issues involved in conducting a multisite clinical trial).

Organizational structure

Key players: the Project MATCH Research Group

Responsibility for planning and conducting the trial was shared by investigators representing the funding agency (NIAAA), the project's Coordinating Center (CC), and the performance sites, or Clinical Research Units (CRUs). Collectively, the 23 investigators representing the NIAAA, the CC, and the CRUs comprised the Project MATCH Research Group, which bore responsibility for conducting the trial and reporting the findings (see Appendix for a complete list of names and institutions).

Funding Agency

In terms of financial support, NIAAA funded, through separate research grants, a coordinating center and nine performance sites for an initial period of 5 years, followed by continuation grants for 3–5 years. In total, NIAAA provided approximately $28 million in support over the 10-year span of the project. Project staff from NIAAA played an active, collaborative role in the trial that entailed considerably more involvement than is usual in government-sponsored research. In addition, NIAAA supported two consultants who actively participated in the development of the research methodology and in the statistical analyses of the data.

NIAAA convened a panel of alcoholism treatment experts, the Data Safety and Monitoring Board (DSMB), which provided independent oversight of the project. The DSMB was not actively involved in the development or conduct of the trial, but met twice yearly to review methodological procedures, client enrollment and participation (e.g., follow-up rates), and clinical safety issues (e.g., cases withdrawn due to clinical deterioration). One important task of the DSMB was to supervise interim data analyses midway through the data collection phase of the trial to determine whether clients in the three treatment conditions differed in terms of treatment outcome. To minimize any bias that could have resulted from knowledge of preliminary results, these analyses, which were conducted primarily for safety reasons, were performed by an investigator who was not associated with the trial, and the results were made available only to the DSMB and NIAAA.

Coordinating Center

NIAAA funded a CC to provide an organizational core for the project separate from the CRUs. The overall function of the CC was to assure standardization across the performance sites and to facilitate communication. The CC divided its functions into two relatively independent components, with two different sets of investigators at two separate physical locations. One component coordinated aspects of the research protocol (e.g., randomization, research assistant training, data processing and analyses); the second dealt with treatment delivery (e.g., development of treatment manuals, therapist training, treatment process analyses). This division of responsibility accorded well with the backgrounds and strengths of the investigators at the two locations. More importantly, this division of labor minimized the potential for biasing results, provided a model for the research and treatment components of the CRUs, and lent credibility to the promise made to participants that research evaluation data were not to be shared with therapists.

Clinical Research Units

Grants were awarded to nine performance sites located in different parts of the USA. The trial consisted of two parallel matching studies, the Outpatient arm, with clients recruited through advertisements and outpatient treatment agencies, and the Aftercare arm, with participants who received Project MATCH treatment following an episode of inpatient or intensive day-hospital treatment. One of the CRUs, located in Milwaukee, Wisconsin, was both an Outpatient and Aftercare site. Four additional Outpatient CRUs were located in Albuquerque, New Mexico; Buffalo, New York; Farmington, Connecticut; and West Haven, Connecticut. Additional Aftercare sites were in Charleston, South Carolina; Houston, Texas; Providence, Rhode Island; and Seattle, Washington.

   Although there were some minor variations, the staff configurations at the CRUs were similar. In many cases, there were co-investigators in addition to the principal investigator. Paralleling the two components of the CC, the research and treatment functions of the trial were separated at the CRU level. At all sites, a full-time project coordinator supervised the day-to-day activities of therapists and research assistants.

Project management

In most multisite clinical trials, management tends to be centralized in the offices of the study chairman and/or a coordinating center. Project MATCH was unusual in that a Steering Committee (SC), composed of funded investigators and NIAAA representatives, managed the trial in close collaboration with the CC. The role of this committee evolved as the trial moved through different phases of the research process. During the initial planning stage, the SC developed the research design and methods, and established policies for the conduct of the trial. During the implementation phase, the SC monitored the progress of the trial and established new policies as needed (e.g., data sharing, publications).

Because the SC met only four times per year, an Executive Committee (EC) was formed from members of the SC to monitor the trial on a more frequent basis. The EC, which met weekly by conference call, included elected representatives from the Outpatient and Aftercare CRUs, as well as a representative from the CC and NIAAA. Depending on the phase of the trial, additional members were appointed to the EC as needed (e.g., a statistician when the analyses testing the primary matching hypotheses were conducted). A major task of the EC was to monitor key performance indicators (e.g., participant enrollment, treatment compliance, follow-up rates), using a tracking procedure that had been implemented by the CC to monitor each client's status in the trial.

In addition to the SC and the EC, several long-term committees and *ad hoc* working groups were established to review materials and formulate proposals regarding trial methodology and policies. These groups provided the major mechanism through which the management tasks of the trial were accomplished. Standing committees focused on assessment, research design, publications, and treatment interventions. Working groups focused on such issues as the influence of therapist characteristics on treatment outcome and the development of data-sharing policies. Committees and working groups met regularly at SC meetings and via conference calls.

Communication and coordination

Communication was critical for implementing a uniform protocol that reflected the decisions made by the trial's SC and for dealing with any problems that arose in the course of conducting the trial. The centralization of all communication through the CC avoided duplication of effort and ensured that everyone associated with the trial received the same information. Communication among investigators was facilitated by the circulation of position papers, proposals, performance indicator data, and other materials. Quarterly SC meetings, weekly EC conference calls, and regular committee conference calls provided additional opportunities for communication and coordination.

A second level of communication was between the trial's CC and the CRUs. The CC centralized communications, distributing the official versions of forms, protocols, and policies. In addition to communicating with staff at each of the CRUs, the CC convened regular conference calls for the project coordinators at the CRUs and sponsored two common training seminars. CC staff also conducted annual site visits to each CRU to assure adherence to the common protocol and to provide an opportunity for more direct communication with the research and treatment staff at each site.

Research design

Two parallel studies

Project MATCH consisted of two parallel studies that differed in terms of their recruitment methods, the treatment stage of study participants, and client characteristics. Clients in the Outpatient arm of the trial were recruited directly from the community or from outpatient treatment centers. In the Aftercare arm, the Project MATCH treatments were offered to clients after they had completed an inpatient or intensive day-hospital treatment. Inclusion criteria required that Outpatient clients had not received any alcohol or mental health treatment in the 90-day period prior to enrollment, whereas Aftercare participants were required to have successfully completed a rehabilitation program. It was expected (and subsequently confirmed, see Chapter 5) that participants in the Aftercare study would differ from their Outpatient counterparts in terms of the severity of alcohol dependence and concomitant problems, thereby providing a fuller range of client heterogeneity to test matching hypotheses (albeit within two separate studies).

Following entry into Project MATCH, clients in the two study arms were treated as similarly as possible. The two parallel studies used identical randomization procedures, assessment instruments, treatment protocols, follow-up evaluations, and data analytic techniques. In addition, the same matching hypotheses were tested in both arms of the trial.

The trial was divided into two arms for several reasons. First, the CRUs that were awarded grants were nearly evenly split in terms of their affiliations with outpatient and inpatient treatment facilities. Given the potential differences in the client populations recruited into outpatient and inpatient treatment programs, it was regarded as inappropriate to collapse across the two settings.

Second, the division of the trial into the two study arms provided a replication of the research design, permitting an investigation of client–treatment matching during two stages of the continuum of care identified in Chapter 1 (i.e., 'during the treatment process' and 'following the rehabilitation intervention'). Further, this replication could increase the applicability and generalizability of the findings to current practices in the alcoholism treatment field. The increased use of outpatient services in response to economic pressures in the USA made it important to consider the potential benefits of client–treatment matching in this treatment environment (Institute of Medicine, 1990). Similarly, aftercare is regarded as an important adjunct to successful outcome following a more intensive treatment experience, and there was some empirical evidence suggesting that type of aftercare may interact with client attributes to produce differential treatment outcomes (Ito & Donovan, 1986; Kadden et al., 1989).

Third, the two arms of Project MATCH permitted the testing of matching hypotheses in two samples that collectively offered a broader range of participant characteristics, particularly in terms of the severity of alcohol dependence and other problems, than would have been found in a study limited to one treatment population. In effect, the two arms of the trial allowed the conduct of two investigations rather than one, and thereby increased the number of parameters that could be considered in the research design (Project MATCH Research Group, 1993).

Critical decisions

There are a number of choices that need to be made in designing a treatment matching study. Each choice involves the consideration of advantages and disadvantages, and the Project MATCH SC debated a variety of alternatives before agreeing upon a final research design. The

critical decisions involved whether to randomize participants to treatments, the choice of a matching strategy, the selection of treatments,
whether to use an untreated control group, and the length of the post-
treatment follow-up period.

Random assignment

As outlined in Chapter 1, several research designs are appropriate for the
investigation of treatment matching. In terms of causal inference, the
randomized clinical trial (RCT) represents the strongest research design.
In matching studies, the RCT essentially allows comparison of matched
and mismatched clients, and lends itself to the examination of a wide range
of potential matching attributes.

Matching strategy

From the matching strategies described in Chapter 1, the trial investigators
decided on 'matching guided by theoretically derived hypotheses.' The
rationale for conducting a multisite trial was based on an assessment of
prior matching research and theory, which was deemed sufficiently developed to justify a large-scale investigation. As described in Chapter 6, the *a
priori* hypotheses tested in the trial were based on existing theory and
accumulated empirical evidence. The matching strategy adopted for the
study would thus contribute not only to clinical practice, but also to an
understanding of the mechanisms that underlie successful treatment
matching.

Treatment selection

The choice of particular interventions for use in the trial necessitated
decisions regarding the type (psychosocial versus pharmacotherapy) as
well as the number and content of the treatments that would be delivered.
   Although a number of pharmacological agents have shown promising
results in alcoholism treatment, such agents are typically used as adjuncts
to other forms of intervention (Kranzler, 2000) rather than as the primary
or exclusive mode of treatment. Further, there are methodological issues
involved in adding an active drug condition to other therapies. These
include the need for a placebo comparison group and, as a consequence, a
doubling of sample size. Administration of a pharmacological agent also
requires involvement of medical staff and further restricts the sample

population by excluding potential participants who are unable to take the drug. Finally, the theoretical and empirical bases for the development of specific matching hypotheses are relatively limited. These considerations led the trial investigators to focus on psychosocial modes of treatment (see also Donovan et al., 1994).

One of the most critical decisions in the trial concerned treatment content. As described more fully in Chapter 4, several criteria were used to select the therapies adopted in Project MATCH: empirical evidence of clinical efficacy; potential for client–treatment matching; applicability within existing treatment systems; specifiable, measurable, and distinct therapeutic ingredients; and feasibility of implementation (cf. Donovan et al., 1994).

Practical (e.g., recruitment feasibility) and methodological (e.g., statistical power) considerations suggested that no more than three treatments could realistically be included in the trial. A number of potential approaches were eliminated for practical reasons (e.g., family therapy), leaving five viable candidates for consideration: Community Reinforcement Approach, Cognitive–Behavioral Therapy (CBT), Motivational Enhancement Therapy (MET), Twelve Step Facilitation (TSF), and Interactional Therapy. Each of the five treatments was formally evaluated using the selection criteria. Although no treatment approach fully satisfied all of the criteria, the three therapies that were most successful were CBT, MET, and TSF.

The CBT was grounded in social learning theory, and was designed to help the client overcome skills deficits and cope with situations that tend to precipitate relapse. The TSF was based on the concept of alcoholism as a spiritual and medical disease. Participants in this therapy were encouraged to develop a commitment to Alcoholics Anonymous (AA) and to work through the Twelve Steps of AA. The MET was rooted in the principles of motivational psychology and focused on producing behavioral change that was internally motivated. All three treatments were delivered over a 12-week period. Whereas CBT and TSF both consisted of weekly therapy sessions, MET involved four sessions, occurring during the first, second, sixth, and twelfth weeks of the treatment period (see Chapter 4 for more detail).

Absence of an untreated control group

Project MATCH did not include an assessment-only, untreated control group, a decision that accorded well with the overall rationale for the trial.

A distinction has been made between traditional 'main effects' treatment outcome research and matching research (DiClemente et al., 1992). Investigations of treatment matching differ considerably from traditional treatment outcome studies in their underlying assumptions. The main effects approach is aimed at demonstrating the relative efficacy of particular treatments relative to a comparison intervention. Minimal-contact comparison groups or placebo-control groups are used to show that the treatment of interest produces therapeutic benefits beyond the influence of nonspecific factors such as attention or assessment.

Matching research is conducted under different circumstances. It is most appropriate when (1) there is no evidence for the superiority of a particular treatment for all individuals with a given condition; (2) there are a number of treatments that appear to be comparable in their effectiveness for undifferentiated participant groups; and (3) there is evidence, within or across treatments, that subsets of individuals differentially benefit. Thus, matching trials involve the use of multiple active treatments that are relatively comparable in terms of outcome for undifferentiated samples. In contrast to the main effects approach, which is aimed at demonstrating the efficacy of a particular intervention, the use of treatments with demonstrated efficacy reduces the need for an untreated control group. Eligibility criteria are designed to promote sample heterogeneity rather than homogeneity. Instead of evaluating main effects via direct treatment comparisons, 'matched' clients are essentially compared with 'mismatched' or 'unmatched' clients. That is, the focus of evaluation is on differential treatment response, reflecting an interaction between client characteristics and the different interventions (cf. Donovan et al., 1994).

Two additional factors influenced the decision to limit the trial to active treatment conditions. First, compared with simple main effects, larger sample sizes are required to achieve adequate statistical power for the detection of the interaction effects that are used to evaluate matching hypotheses. Thus, the sample size requirement for the trial was already large; inclusion of an untreated control group would have required the recruitment of still more participants, a task that did not seem feasible. Second, ethical considerations mitigated against the use of an untreated control group; to deny treatments of proven effectiveness to people with severe alcohol dependence is unethical.

Follow-up evaluations

In considering the overall design of the trial, investigators debated the number and timing of follow-up evaluations. Frequent assessment sessions have the advantage of producing more information about the course of treatment response, and they may facilitate continued research participation because it is easier to locate clients when the intervals between evaluations are short. Frequent outcome assessments carried out over an extended period also permit greater flexibility in comparing results with other studies. On the other hand, frequent follow-up sessions increase the potential for the assessment itself to influence outcome, and place an added burden on clients in terms of time and effort, which may contribute to participant attrition.

In attempting to balance these issues, the design included five follow-up evaluations conducted at 3-month intervals, commencing at the end of the 12-week treatment period and ending 1 year later. Three months represented a time frame for which events should remain relatively salient in memory, and the contacts were sufficiently frequent for client-tracking purposes. This schedule of follow-up evaluations also accorded well with other investigations of treatment outcome, which tend to report results 6 or 12 months following treatment. To ease the burden on participants, and to reduce the potential effects of assessment *per se*, two of the sessions were quite brief, focusing primarily on drinking behavior during the assessment period, and one of these was conducted by telephone. The remaining sessions were more comprehensive, including collateral informant interviews and the collection of blood and urine specimens.

To assess the long-term effects of treatment and the durability of treatment matches, a 3-year follow-up (39 months following the initiation of treatment) was conducted for clients in the Outpatient arm of the trial. Resources did not permit the conduct of a long-term follow-up evaluation in the Aftercare sample.

Overview of client participation

The final research design is depicted graphically in Figure 2.1, which presents a flow chart illustrating a typical client's progress through the trial. First, potential clients were initially screened for eligibility. There were slight differences in inclusion/exclusion criteria for Outpatient and Aftercare participants. If individuals appeared to meet selection criteria,

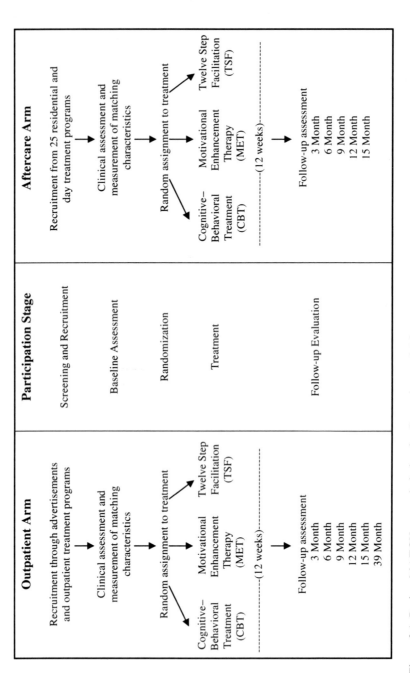

Figure 2.1 Project MATCH research design for Outpatient and Aftercare arms.

informed consent was obtained, and they were enrolled in the trial. Participants completed a comprehensive baseline assessment battery during three intake sessions (the Diagnostic Interview, the Pre-treatment Evaluation, and the Psychological Evaluation). Eligibility criteria were reviewed following the second of these sessions, and clients were randomized to one of the three treatments. Following a 12-week treatment regimen, they entered the follow-up phase of the trial, during which they completed five interviews over a 12-month period. Outpatient clients also participated in a long-term (3-year) follow-up evaluation.

Summary

This chapter provides a description of the basic organizational structure of Project MATCH and an overview of the research design. Decision making during the trial was shared by CC and CRU investigators, who worked in concert with NIAAA staff and consultants. In addition to the basic decisions regarding research design, the investigators were confronted with additional dilemmas as they considered the eligibility criteria for the two arms of the trial, developed the assessment battery, and planned the delivery of treatment. The nature of the choices, the criteria employed in making them, and the compromises that were reached are discussed in the three chapters that follow. What is not discussed in these chapters are the human and social elements of collaborative research, which constitute an unwritten story behind a scientific project that is often as interesting as the formal research report. Project MATCH was designed after the investigators were chosen, based on research proposals that were submitted by 10 Principal Investigators who were competing with a larger group of applicants. Once the investigators had been selected, they were asked to put aside their research proposals and work together to develop a common protocol that would address the key goals of the project. Drawing from the expertise of the different investigators, who represented psychiatry, psychology, and other disciplines, and the ideas contained in their individual proposals, the Project MATCH Research Group spent a full year discussing, debating, and compromising until a coherent research design emerged that suited the needs of the NIAAA and the preferences of the investigators. In the course of this process, it became evident that science is a social, as well as a rational, enterprise. The debates over treatments, recruitment settings, assessment procedures, and matching hypotheses were all influenced by investigator differences in personalities, working styles, ideological preferences, and professional experience, but the process developed by the Project MATCH Research Group, one that required reasoned argument and majority rule, in the end resulted in a research plan that was far better than the sum of the individual research proposals that initially qualified the investigators for their place on the Steering Committee. Within this organizational model, the Coordinating Center served at times as a facilitator, at times as a leader, and at times as mediator and arbitrator, but it always served the will of the Steering Committee. Although the decision-making process in the design of large-scale research projects is rarely discussed in terms of its personal and social dimensions, Project MATCH proved that cooperative agreement is an effective mechanism for funding and managing a multisite study.

3

Clinical assessment: measuring matching characteristics and treatment outcomes

GERARD J. CONNORS, WILLIAM R. MILLER, RAYMOND F. ANTON, AND J. SCOTT TONIGAN

Clinical assessment plays a vital role in the evaluation of treatment matching. In the case of Project MATCH, the assessment procedures were used to screen research volunteers for study inclusion, provide a clinical description of the study participants, assess matching attributes, and measure treatment outcomes. This chapter describes the criteria used to select measures, the sequencing and administration of the assessment battery, the instruments that comprised the battery, and the methodological and practical considerations involved in its administration.

Screening for study inclusion

An important requirement of clinical research is to identify a client population that is appropriate for both the treatment and research protocols. Inclusion and exclusion criteria are developed for this purpose. In general, the clients to be included are those for whom the treatment or treatments are expected to hold potential benefit. When clients are excluded, it typically is because the treatment is not considered appropriate for their particular circumstances, or because of personal or logistic impediments that preclude participation. For example, an alcohol-abusing client who is acutely psychotic or suicidal may require the kind of immediate attention that is not part of a particular treatment protocol. Other clients may be ineligible because they live a considerable distance from the treatment site or because of unstable living circumstances that could interfere with their ability to attend treatment sessions. The inclusion and exclusion criteria for Project MATCH were developed on the basis of these considerations (Project MATCH Research Group, 1993).

The inclusion criteria for the Outpatient arm were a current diagnosis of alcohol abuse or dependence according to the *Diagnostic and Statistical*

Manual, 3rd edition, revised (DSM-III-R; American Psychiatric Association, 1987); alcohol as the principal drug of abuse; active drinking during the 3 months prior to study enrollment; minimum age of 18 years; and minimum sixth-grade reading level. Exclusion criteria were a DSM-III-R diagnosis of current dependence on sedative/hypnotic drugs, stimulants, cocaine or opiates; any intravenous drug use in the prior 6 months; currently a danger to self or others; probation/parole requirements that might interfere with protocol participation; residential instability; inability to identify at least one person to assist with locating the client for follow-up assessments; acute psychosis; severe organic impairment; and involvement in an alternative treatment for alcohol-related problems other than that provided by Project MATCH. Regarding the last exclusion criterion, involvement was defined as more than 6 hours of nonstudy treatment, except for participation in self-help groups such as Alcoholics Anonymous.

The inclusion criteria for the Aftercare arm of the study were similar, with the following modifications: DSM-III-R symptoms of alcohol abuse or dependence and requisite drinking behavior were assessed for the 3 months prior to an inpatient or day-hospital admission; completion of a program of at least 7 days of inpatient or intensive day-hospital treatment (not including detoxification); and referral for aftercare by the inpatient or day-hospital treatment staff.

Several other general admission requirements applied to all participants: a willingness to accept randomization to any of the three treatment conditions; residence within a reasonable commuting distance, with available transportation to treatment and assessment sessions; and completion of prior detoxification when medically indicated.

The development of these selection criteria reflects a complex decision-making process (see Zweben et al., 1994). A primary concern was to recruit participants appropriate for testing the primary and secondary matching hypotheses. The eligibility criteria needed to be broad enough to ensure sufficient diversity within the sample on the various client characteristics to be evaluated.

Measuring client prognostic variables and matching attributes

In addition to screening for eligibility, the development of the assessment battery also included consideration of both prognostic and matching variables. Prognostic variables are factors that influence outcomes equally across the treatment conditions being evaluated. Examples of prognostic variables include age, occupational status, education, and drinking history. These 'main effect' predictor variables are often used as covariates in statistical analyses.

Matching variables, on the other hand, are attributes that differentially influence treatment outcomes across the treatment conditions being evaluated. In an investigation of client–treatment matching, the specification and measurement of matching variables are among the most crucial assessment issues to be addressed. Given their importance, particular care is needed to select matching variables for which reliable and valid measures exist.

Whereas a number of demographic factors and drinking history variables can be assessed directly through the use of simple questions or clinical records, many other variables must be assessed using validated psychometric instruments. Examples of such instruments used in Project MATCH include the Alcohol Use Inventory (AUI: Wanberg, Horn, & Foster, 1977) to assess alcohol involvement; the University of Rhode Island Change Assessment instrument (URICA: DiClemente & Hughes, 1990) to measure motivational readiness to change; the socialization scale of the California Personality Inventory (CPI: Gough, 1975) to assess sociopathy; and the psychiatric severity section of the Addiction Severity Index (ASI: McLellan et al., 1980) to evaluate psychiatric impairment.

There are occasions when no definitive or widely accepted test has been developed to measure a client attribute. In this case, multiple measures of the variable are often used to create a single composite score to represent the construct in question. This approach was used in several cases. Cognitive impairment, for example, was represented by performance on the Shipley Institute of Living Scale (Shipley, 1946) and the Symbol–Digit Modalities Test (Smith, 1973). Another example concerns alcoholic typology. The composite typology index used in Project MATCH classified clients as Type B alcoholics, representing high vulnerability and high severity of alcoholism, or as Type A, reflecting low vulnerability and severity, based on scores derived from five different instruments (see Chapter 6).

Measuring treatment outcomes

It is critical in any study of treatment matching to conduct a comprehensive assessment of multiple dimensions of client functioning, because different treatments have the potential to influence different aspects of outcome, ranging from drinking behavior to employment functioning. Accordingly, it is important to gather follow-up data reflecting outcomes that are likely to be influenced by each treatment, as well as by alcoholism treatment in general. Moreover, if matching effects are found, questions arise regarding the strength and robustness of the findings. Does matching affect the amount and pattern of drinking? Does it facilitate psychosocial adjustment? Do various effects endure over time? Conversely, do unmatched individuals do worse in specific outcome domains? All of these questions demand multiple outcome criteria.

Difficult choices were made in the selection of outcome variables. Even the most obvious outcome in alcoholism treatment, alcohol consumption, can be measured in a variety of ways and from different perspectives (Babor et al., 1994). Total abstinence rate, latency to relapse, amount consumed on specific occasions, heavy drinking days, drinking with consequences, patterns of consumption, blood alcohol concentration (BAC) estimates, and average consumption over specified time periods have all been used as outcome variables in alcoholism treatment research. Constructs related to consumption, such as sobriety, 'slip,' lapse, and relapse, represent another level of complexity. Drinking-related consequences are additional areas of functioning that can be assessed in order to obtain a comprehensive view of outcome, along with personal and social functioning (Moos et al., 1990).

The use of multiple outcome measures must be weighed against the risk of Type 1 error (i.e., the possibility of finding a statistically significant result by chance because many variables are tested). To resolve this dilemma, the investigators assessed a wide variety of potential outcome variables, but selected two primary outcome measures for the formal evaluation of all study hypotheses. The first was Percent Days Abstinent (PDA), which provided a measure of drinking frequency; the second was Drinks per Drinking Day (DDD), which constituted a measure of drinking intensity. The selection of these two primary outcome variables was guided in large part by the need to have relevant indicators of alcohol consumption that were somewhat independent (Babor et al., 1994).

In addition to these primary dimensions of outcome, a variety of supplemental outcome variables were assessed. These included negative consequences associated with drinking, biological indicators of drinking – including serum gamma-glutamyl transpeptidase (GGTP) and carbohydrate-deficient transferrin (CDT) (Anton & Moak, 1994) –

measures of subsequent treatment utilization, and measures of other life-functioning domains (e.g., employment status, mood/affect).

Based on the recognition that single measures of alcohol use and related problems cannot capture the full range of experiences resulting from participation in treatment (Duckitt et al., 1985), a composite outcome measure was also developed. Empirical evidence indicates that individuals may have differing levels of alcohol problem severity despite having similar consumption patterns (Zweben & Cisler, 1996). Using conceptually driven criteria for alcohol use and related consequences, individuals were assigned to one of four composite categories at intake, and again at each of the five follow-up points: (1) abstinent; (2) moderate drinking without problems; (3) heavy drinking *or* recurring alcohol problems; and (4) heavy drinking and recurring problems.

Criteria for instrument selection

A comprehensive set of measures was assembled for administration at intake, during the treatment phase, and at each of the post-treatment follow-up evaluations. The baseline battery consisted of three separate assessment sessions (excluding the initial screening interview) requiring a total of approximately 6–8 hours to complete. Assessment procedures were varied, including personal interviews, computer-assisted instruments, self-administered questionnaires, and biochemical assays. The following guidelines were used to select the assessments.

- *Measurement of a wide range of potential matching variables.* Because the goal of Project MATCH was to study client–treatment interaction effects, efforts were made to measure as many potentially relevant matching variables as possible.
- *Measurement of characteristics relevant to* a priori *matching hypotheses.* Selection of matching and outcome assessments was guided by the nature of the treatments and the matching hypotheses under evaluation. For example, with the emphasis on a 'higher power' in the Twelve Step Facilitation intervention, one of the three treatments under investigation (see Chapter 4), the trial would have been remiss not to include some measure of spirituality or religiosity.
- *Adoption of standard, widely used assessment instruments.* Whenever possible, preference was given to instruments used in prior alcoholism treatment or matching research (Mattson et al., 1994; Allen &

Columbus, 1995). The primary intent of this guideline was to facilitate the comparison of findings between Project MATCH and other studies. In some cases, there were no standard measures that would meet the project's needs. In such cases, instruments were revised or newly created, such as the Form-90 drinking assessment instrument (Miller & Del Boca, 1994), the Drinker Inventory of Consequences (Miller et al., 1995b), and the Important People and Activities interview (Clifford & Longabaugh, 1991). Fortunately, the large and diverse sample of participants in Project MATCH allowed extensive evaluation of the psychometric properties of newly constructed or adapted measures.

- *Use of instruments with acceptable psychometric properties.* Reliability, scaling properties, validity, and response distribution considerations were central to the selection process.
- *Corroboration of verbal reports.* Although self-reports of alcohol use and related problems have been shown to be reliable and valid when data collection conditions are optimally structured (Babor et al., 1990; Del Boca & Noll, 2000), several independent data sources were used to corroborate verbal reports. In addition to providing information regarding the physical consequences of alcohol consumption, liver enzyme tests were used to evaluate self-reports of drinking (Anton & Moak, 1994). Urinanalyses provided an alternative source of information regarding illicit drug use, and collateral informant interviews served as an independent data source regarding alcohol use, treatment experiences, and other life events assessed with the Form-90 client interview.

The Project MATCH assessment battery

Prospective study participants were screened initially using the Quick Screen interview that collected basic demographic and clinical information relevant to the inclusion/exclusion criteria. Clients eligible for further evaluation were then scheduled for a Diagnostic Evaluation session. This in turn was followed by a Pretreatment Evaluation session and a Psychological Evaluation session. Many of the instruments administered at baseline were also completed during follow-up evaluations. Scores derived from these assessments were used as secondary outcome measures or as intervening variables that might explain the causal chains behind the *a priori* matching hypotheses.

The assessment battery is summarized in Table 3.1. The measures are categorized into eight domains: alcohol involvement, psychological/psychiatric functioning, social support, spirituality, neuropsychological status, biological functioning, collateral informant reports, and therapy process. Listed within each domain are the variables derived from each measure. In the following pages, variable names are capitalized when they refer to a specific measure (e.g., Motivation as measured by the URICA) and are listed in lower case (e.g., motivation) when referring to the more generic construct.

The alcohol involvement measures were designed to provide information on lifetime and recent drinking, consequences of alcohol use, and nature and extent of alcohol involvement. As shown in Table 3.1, alcohol diagnoses and alcohol involvement were assessed by instruments that have been widely used in treatment research. The instrument from which the two primary drinking outcome measures (PDA and DDD) were computed, the Form-90, was developed specifically for use in Project MATCH. The Form-90 is a family of structured interviews designed for detailed assessment of drinking behavior during a time window of approximately 90 days. The core interview is a hybrid of two existing instruments – the Time Line Follow Back (Sobell & Sobell, 1992) and the Comprehensive Drinker Profile (Miller & Marlatt, 1984) – and uses aided-recall techniques to generate a daily record of alcohol consumption for the entire follow-up period (Miller & Del Boca, 1994; Miller, 1996).

Psychological functioning was assessed in terms of affective disorders, anxiety disorders, anger, sociopathy, antisocial personality disorder, and general psychiatric impairment. In addition, this domain included measures of motivational readiness to change drinking behavior, and confidence (self-efficacy) to achieve alcohol abstinence. The social support category included assessment of important people in the person's life and their support for the client's drinking, the work-place environment, and involvement in Alcoholics Anonymous. Spirituality is an elusive concept considered particularly relevant to the evaluation of an intervention based on a Twelve Step model. This domain was assessed using measures of purpose in life, the seeking of transcendent goals in life, and religious beliefs and behaviors. Neuropsychological functioning was measured using well-established tests, including the Shipley Institute of Living Scale and the Symbol–Digit Modalities Test. Blood tests were conducted to assess liver functioning, and CDT served as a marker for recent alcohol consumption. Urine samples were collected to measure other drug use, and breathalyzer instruments were used to determine the client's BAC prior to

Table 3.1. *The Project MATCH assessment battery*

Assessment domain/ variable name	Measure[a]	Source documents
Alcohol involvement		
Dependence diagnosis	Structured Clinical Interview for DSM-III-R (SCID) (alcohol, drug sections)[b]	Spitzer & Williams (1985)
Percent days abstinent, drinks per drinking day	Form 90[c]	Miller (1996)
Alcohol-related consequences	Drinker Inventory of Consequences (DrInC)[b]	Miller et al. (1995b)
Alcohol involvement	Alcohol Use Inventory (AUI)[c]	Wanberg et al. (1977)
Psychological/psychiatric functioning		
Psychotic symptoms	SCID Psychotic Screen[b]	Spitzer & Williams (1985)
Psychiatric severity	Addiction Severity Index[b]	McLellan et al. (1992)
Affective disorders, anxiety disorders, antisocial personality disorder	Computerized Diagnostic Interview Schedule (C-DIS)[d]	Robins et al. (1981); Blouin et al. (1988)
Depression	Beck Depression Inventory[d]	Beck et al. (1961)
Anger	State–Trait Anger Scale[d]	Spielberger et al. (1983)
Sociopathy	California Psychological Inventory – Socialization Scale[b]	Gough (1975, 1987)
Temptation to drink and confidence to abstain	Alcohol Abstinence Self-efficacy (AASE) scale[c]	DiClemente (1986); DiClemente et al. (1994a)
Motivation to change	University of Rhode Island Change Assessment (URICA)[b]	DiClemente & Hughes (1990); Prochaska & DiClemente (1992)
Readiness to change	Stages of Change Readiness and Treatment Eagerness Scale (SOCRATES)[b]	Miller & Tonigan (1996)
Conceptual level	Paragraph completion test[d]	Hunt et al. (1978)
Interpersonal dependency	Interpersonal Dependency Inventory – Assertion of Autonomy Scale[c]	Hirschfeld et al. (1977)
	Personal Attributes Questionnaire[c]	Spence et al. (1974)
Impulsivity	Differential Personality Questionnaire Control versus Impulsivity Subscale[d]	Tellegen (1982)
Social support		
Support for drinking	Important People and Activities (IPA) Instrument[d]	Clifford & Longabaugh (1991)
	Your Work Place[c]	Beattie et al. (1992)

	Social Support Questionnaire (friends and family forms)[e]	Procidano & Heller (1983)
Positive social support	AA Involvement Scale[b]	Tonigan et al. (1996a)
Involvement in Alcoholics Anonymous		
Psychosocial functioning	Psychosocial Functioning Inventory[c]	Feragne et al. (1983)
Spirituality		
Current life meaning	Purpose in Life Scale[b]	Crumbaugh & Maholick (1976)
Desire for greater life meaning	Seeking of Noetic Goals Scale[b]	Crumbaugh (1977a, 1977b)
Religious involvement	Religious Background and Beliefs[b]	Connors et al. (1996)
Neuropsychological status		
Cognitive impairment	Shipley Institute of Living Abstraction Scale[c]	Shipley (1946)
	Trailmaking Test Parts A and B[c]	Reitan (1958)
	Symbol Digit Modalities Test[c]	Smith (1973)
Biological functioning		
Liver function tests	GGTP, ASAT, ALAT[b]	Anton & Moak (1994)
	Carbohydrate-deficient transferrin[b]	Anton & Moak (1994)
Drug/alcohol use	Urine toxicology,[b,e] Breathalyzer tests[b]	
Collateral informant reports		
Client drinking	Form-90 – Collateral Version	Miller (1996)
Therapy process[f]		
Perceptions of therapy	Therapist and Patient Session Rating Forms	Carroll et al. (1994, 1998)
Client/therapist relationship	Working Alliance Inventory	Horvath & Greenberg (1986)

[a]Some measures were modified for use in Project MATCH, and several were developed specifically for use in this trial. The majority of these measures were re-administered at some or all of the follow-up evaluations.
[b]Measure administered during the Diagnostic Evaluation, the first assessment session.
[c]Measure administered during the Pre-treatment Evaluation, the second assessment session.
[d]Measure administered during the Psychological Evaluation, the third assessment session.
[e]Urine toxicologies were used for assessment of opiates, cannabinoids, amphetamines, benzodiazepines, and cocaine.
[f]Process assessments are described in greater detail in Chapter 10.
GGTP, serum gamma-glutamyl transpeptidase; ASAT, serum aspartate aminotransferase; ALAT, serum alanine aminotransferase.

treatment and assessment sessions. In addition, interviews were conducted with a collateral informant, such as a friend or family member, to obtain another perspective on the client's alcohol use. Finally, process assessments were conducted during the treatment phase of the project to measure the therapeutic alliance from the perspectives of both the client and the therapist.

It is important to emphasize that the assessment battery was developed to meet the general requirements of a client–treatment matching study as well as the specific needs of the hypotheses being evaluated in this trial. Whereas this battery might be useful in whole or in part in research and clinical applications of client–treatment matching, appropriate modifications would be warranted to meet the needs and objectives of those endeavors.

Issues in the administration of assessment instruments

A major challenge was to develop an assessment protocol that appeared from the client's perspective to be meaningful and integrated, but that at the same time maximized the validity of protracted assessments. The validity of data collection may be compromised by assessment reactivity, potential order effects, and sensitivity of measurement to recent alcohol consumption. Practical issues of timing and sequencing of assessments include task demands, detecting and managing clients who are under the influence of alcohol, and responsiveness of the protocol to the requirements of the research design.

Methodological considerations

An important consideration in this context is assessment reactivity, which reflects the altering of a client attribute (e.g., drinking or motivation for treatment) as a function of its measurement. Assessment reactivity is most commonly considered in terms of its impact on the main effect of the intervention. For example, comprehensive measurement of alcohol consumption may alter subsequent alcohol use because the assessment heightened the client's awareness of the severity of drinking. In matching studies, reactivity is especially important because of the potential for 'interactive reactivity,' whereby measurement of one client matching attribute covaries with changes in other attributes also hypothesized to produce differential outcomes across treatments. In contrast to measurement order effects, which are systematic *across* individuals, inter-active reactivity may occur only in certain clients. The more that predictor variables or predictor and outcome variables covary, the greater the risk of interactive reactivity.

To minimize these problems, it was decided to schedule instruments with the highest likelihood of assessment reactivity early in the assessment process. For example, motivation to change drinking behavior had signifi-cant potential to increase with continued involvement in the assessment process. Consequently, measurement of this domain was placed in the first assessment session. In contrast, other variables were deemed more resilient to interactive reactivity effects, and were scheduled later. These included social support, conceptual level, and antisocial personality disorder.

In matching studies, order effects may be considered as a subset of interactive reactivity. Order effects are most likely to occur with invariant sequencing of self-report questionnaires, although they can also arise in connection with structured interviews. The greater the overlap in the content of two adjacent questionnaires, the higher the probability that an order effect will be produced. Two strategies were employed to counteract this potential confounding effect. First, the initial sequencing of question-naires was randomized and then re-sequenced such that the first question-naire for the first client became the second questionnaire for the second client, and so forth. Second, because it was felt that this strategy did not sufficiently reduce the potential for carry-over effects, particularly with respect to the assessment of alcohol involvement, similar measures (e.g., the Alcohol Use Inventory and the Drinker Inventory of Consequences) were administered at different points in the assessment process.

Another important issue in sequencing instruments involves sensitivity of the measurement to recent alcohol consumption. For biological assess-ments (e.g., blood and urine), optimal timing depends on how the informa-tion will be used. If liver function tests are used to corroborate self-reported baseline drinking, samples should be drawn before or soon after cessation of drinking. However, if the initial liver function measures are used to provide a non-drinking baseline for comparison to follow-up tests, samples should be drawn several weeks after initial cessation of drinking. Sense of purpose in life and motivation to stop drinking are probably best measured early in the assessment sequence. On the other hand, excessive alcohol consumption is known to elevate depression and confound assess-ment of psychiatric disorders. As a result, the psychiatric assessments occurred at the end of the baseline assessment phase.

Practical considerations

Two practical issues were considered in relation to the use of such a lengthy assessment battery: (1) the effect of the assessment on the accuracy of information, and (2) the possibility that the assessment alone influenced outcomes. Each of these issues affected the ultimate sequencing of the battery.

Concern about client fatigue resulted in the decision to limit each assessment session to roughly 2 hours. Each instrument placed different demands upon participants. Some demanded accurate recall (e.g., Form-90) and others required the use of abstraction abilities (e.g., the neuropsychological battery). Thus, the arrangement of instruments within assessment periods was varied to avoid overtaxing a particular client's ability to respond.

An issue that arises when conducting an extensive assessment battery is the potential effect that the assessment itself might have on outcome. It could be argued that the assessments *per se* are therapeutic and might well contribute positively to outcome. Alternatively, one also could argue that the burden of assessment might overwhelm the client or that the assessments might not be viewed as relevant, leading to withdrawal from treatment and poorer overall outcomes. To minimize the chances of either of these effects, the intake assessment battery was conducted in a manner that was integrated with the treatment clients received. Although it was made clear that neither the type nor the duration of treatment was contingent upon participants' responses, there was a greater chance that clients would feel they were receiving a thorough diagnostic evaluation that had some relevance to treatment. At the same time, the independence of the research and treatment components was emphasized to reduce the possibility that participants would minimize their drinking in follow-up evaluations in order to present a more favorable image to their therapists.

It was assumed that clients whose BAC exceeded 0.10 would not provide reliable and valid data. As a result, all intake and follow-up interviews began with a breath test. Clients with BACs exceeding 0.10 were rescheduled for a later appointment. Discretion was left to interviewers to terminate the assessment session in instances when the BAC was between 0.05 and 0.10.

Another practical issue was the need to confirm the accuracy of certain types of data while the client was still in the assessment process. Data collected early in the assessment process included identification of a client 'locator' to assist research staff in finding clients at follow-up. Efforts were made to identify two collateral informants to be interviewed at intake and follow-up. When locators or collateral informants could not be contacted, research assistants encouraged clients to provide additional names. Other data required early in the assessment sequence were the information needed for the urn randomization procedure (e.g., age, gender, years of education, marital status, dependence severity, and employment status: see Chapter 5) and for the first session of Motivational Enhancement Therapy (see Chapter 4) when clients were provided with individualized feedback about their drinking and its negative consequences.

Summary

The formulation of the client assessment battery is among the most challenging tasks facing clinical researchers planning a study on client–treatment matching. Fortunately, significant progress has been made in the development and validation of a wide variety of clinical assessments that can be used to measure matching characteristics and treatment outcomes. The application of these measures to the research objectives of Project MATCH made it possible to conduct a comprehensive test of the matching hypotheses.

4

Therapies for matching: selection, development, implementation, and costs

DENNIS M. DONOVAN, KATHLEEN M. CARROLL,
RONALD M. KADDEN, CARLO C. DICLEMENTE,
AND BRUCE J. ROUNSAVILLE

A variety of different treatments were considered for use in Project MATCH and three interventions were chosen: Cognitive–Behavioral Therapy (CBT), Motivational Enhancement Therapy (MET), and Twelve Step Facilitation (TSF). This chapter describes the three treatments; the selection, training, supervision, and monitoring of 80 therapists; the evaluation of the interventions in terms of their integrity and discriminability; procedures for dealing with clinically deteriorated clients; and the costs involved in treatment delivery. Session attendance for all three manualized treatments, which were delivered as individual therapy over a 12-week period, was excellent. Ratings of session videotapes indicated a high degree of treatment integrity and discriminability.

The possibility that matching can improve outcomes is considered when there are a number of treatments with demonstrated efficacy that are comparable in their effectiveness. A second condition is evidence of differential outcome either within or across treatments for subtypes of clients (Miller, 1989b; Lindström, 1992; Donovan et al., 1994). The recognition that these considerations were applicable to existing treatments for alcohol dependence set the stage for the process of selecting, implementing, and evaluating the therapies employed in Project MATCH (Carroll et al., 1994; Donovan et al., 1994).

Selection of therapies

Criteria used to choose therapies

The large variety of available treatment alternatives made the selection of therapies a difficult choice. To assist the selection process, the investigators developed a set of criteria to be used in evaluating potential therapies.

These criteria specified that the therapies should:

1. have prior documentation of clinical effectiveness;
2. have evidence of, or a strong theoretical rationale for, an interaction between the treatment and some client characteristic;
3. be relevant to the needs of a broad range of individuals with alcohol problems;
4. be acceptable to practitioners in the treatment community;
5. have active therapeutic ingredients that are specifiable, measurable, and distinct from other treatments in their mechanisms of action;
6. be feasible to implement within the methodological constraints of a clinical trial (Donovan et al., 1994).

Practical and methodological considerations (e.g., statistical power, client recruitment) dictated that no more than three therapies could be included in the trial. A number of candidate therapies were considered, none of which satisfied all of the criteria. However, three therapies met most of the conditions.

Description of the therapies

The three therapies were a cognitive–behavioral intervention based on social skills and coping skills training approaches (Monti et al., 1989), a brief intervention based on motivational interviewing and enhancement principles (Miller & Rollnick, 1991), and an Alcoholics Anonymous (AA)-oriented Twelve Step Facilitation (TSF) approach (Nowinski & Baker, 1992).

Cognitive–Behavioral Therapy

Of the three therapies selected, Cognitive–Behavioral Therapy (CBT) was the only one that had previously demonstrated differential outcomes based on client–treatment matching (Kadden et al., 1989; Donovan & Marlatt, 1993). Cognitive–behavioral approaches in general, and coping skills training more specifically, derive from social learning theory. It is assumed that the client is deficient in those cognitive, behavioral, and affective skills necessary to deal with problems in a number of life areas. In the absence of such skills, individuals may turn to drinking as a means of trying to cope (e.g., an individual drinks to deal with depression or to enhance sociability). Over time, drinking becomes functionally related to the problems in people's lives as their primary means of coping with them. Given the relationship between alcohol use and problem situations, skills training approaches address the broad spectrum of problems that may be related to drinking, rather than focusing only on the drinking itself. The overall goal of CBT is to enable the client to master those skills necessary to achieve and maintain abstinence from alcohol and other drugs. To achieve this goal, the client identifies high-risk situations that may increase the likelihood of drinking and is assisted in developing active behavioral or cognitive coping methods to deal with them, rather than relying on alcohol as a familiar but maladaptive coping strategy (Chaney, 1989; Monti et al., 1989).

The clinical methods used in CBT incorporate aspects of behavioral and cognitive therapy, relapse prevention techniques, and strategies for enhancing self-efficacy (Donovan & Chaney, 1985). The therapeutic process trains the client to acquire and apply coping skills, using activities such as problem solving, modeling of appropriate behaviors, cognitive and behavioral rehearsal, and role playing. Clients are also given homework assignments or 'practice exercises' that are to be completed between sessions. These exercises provide the opportunity to practice skills in real-life situations. The clinical activities in CBT focus on overcoming skill deficits and increasing the ability to cope with high-risk situations that commonly precipitate relapse, including both interpersonal difficulties (e.g., conflicts) and intrapersonal discomfort such as anger or depression (e.g., Marlatt & Gordon, 1985; Monti et al., 1989).

CBT in Project MATCH was delivered in 12 therapy sessions over a 12-week period. As described in the CBT treatment manual (Kadden et al., 1992a), the intervention was staged, progressing from core to elective sessions. The initial core sessions, which all clients received, focused on drinking-related topics, such as strategies to help achieve sobriety for those in the Outpatient arm of the trial and to prevent relapse among those in the Aftercare arm. The core sessions dealt with understanding the importance of coping skills to prevent relapse, coping with cravings and urges to drink, managing thoughts about alcohol and drinking, developing general problem-solving and drink-refusal skills, dealing with seemingly irrelevant decisions that lead to drinking, and developing plans to cope with relapse if it occurs.

After the seven core sessions, the client and therapist together chose four elective sessions from a menu of 14 alternatives. These sessions dealt with more generalized social, interpersonal, and psychological issues that may lead to drinking, with the goal of developing skills necessary to cope effectively with them. An assumption of CBT is that addressing a broad spectrum of problems is more effective than focusing on drinking alone. The elective topics included nonverbal communication, assertiveness, dealing with criticism, management of anger and negative thoughts, increasing pleasant activities, managing negative moods, expanding social support networks, job-seeking skills, and couples/family issues. Up to two sessions in the elective portion of CBT permitted the participation of a spouse or significant other.

The therapist in CBT was actively involved as both a role model and a teacher of coping skills. Thus, the therapist needed to possess good interpersonal skills in addition to basic clinical knowledge.

Motivational Enhancement Therapy

Increasing attention has been placed on the development and evaluation of brief treatment interventions for use with alcohol-abusing and alcohol-dependent individuals (Institute of Medicine, 1990; Holder et al., 1991). Several forms of brief therapy exist, differing with respect to their duration, content, and goals. Bien et al. (1993) concluded a review of brief interventions by suggesting that outcome evaluations have consistently demonstrated an incremental effect of motivational enhancement interventions over no-treatment control conditions, but with no apparent additional incremental effect over more extensive treatments. It is assumed that brief interventions are more cost effective than lengthier therapies (e.g., Holder et al., 1991).

The specific approach developed for Project MATCH (Miller et al., 1992) had as its primary goal the mobilization of the individual's own resources to bring about the changes needed to achieve sobriety (Miller, 1989a). Unlike CBT, which emphasizes deficits in coping skills, MET assumes that the individual has the requisite skills to successfully recover, but needs encouragement and motivation to put them into action. The primary responsibility for change is believed to lie with the individual. The therapist assumes the role of a collaborator in the change process, providing a therapeutic climate that will enhance the individual's intrinsic motivation to initiate and persist in behavior change efforts. The therapeutic approach is based on the general principles of motivational psychology and behavior change (Miller, 1985; Miller & Rollnick, 1991).

MET incorporates elements found in successful brief intervention strategies with problem drinkers (e.g., Heather, 1989; Miller, 1989a; Miller & Rollnick, 1991). These elements are summarized by the acronym FRAMES: successful interventions are those that provide Feedback regarding personal risk, negative consequences, or impairments related to drinking; place an emphasis on accepting personal Responsibility for change; give clear Advice to change; present a Menu of alternative change options; include an Empathic therapist style; and facilitate the client's Self-efficacy and optimism.

As delivered in Project MATCH, MET consisted of four individual sessions over the 12-week treatment period. The first session was used to provide structured feedback based on pre-treatment assessments of alcohol consumption and related medical, psychological, and social consequences. Feedback was given about the individual's drinking behavior (number of standard drinks per week, and how this compares to adult Americans of the same sex), level of intoxication (estimated blood alcohol concentration (BAC) peaks in a typical week and on one of the heavier days of drinking), risk factors (tolerance level, other drug use, score on the McAndrew Alcoholism Scale, and age of onset of heavy drinking), negative consequences related to drinking, blood tests results (aspartate aminotransferase, SGOT; gamma-glutamyl transpeptidase, GGTP; alanine aminotransferase, SGPT; uric acid; bilirubin), and neuropsychological test performance. The aim of this feedback was to elicit self-motivational statements which reflect increased awareness of the problems associated with drinking, indicate concern about the problem, and evidence a commitment to make behavioral changes. The second session was intended to enhance the commitment to change by asking the individual to develop a more formal plan for behavior change. The worksheet completed with the client focused on specific changes to be made, reasons for changing, steps to be taken to make these changes, people to enlist in the change process, and potential obstacles to overcome. To further increase motivation and gain support for change efforts, attempts were made to involve the client's spouse or significant other in the first two sessions. The last two sessions, held in therapy weeks 6 and 12, monitored the progress the client had made in implementing the change plan, considered barriers encountered in the process, and encouraged continued work toward the specified goals.

Of the three Project MATCH therapies, Motivational Enhancement Therapy (MET) placed the greatest emphasis on therapists' interpersonal and therapeutic style (Miller & Rollnick, 1991). While therapists selected for all three interventions were expected to have general clinical skills, MET therapists had to be reflective and empathic; solicit the client's self-statements about potential problem areas; accentuate the discrepancy between the individual's current behavior and personally important goals and values; avoid or minimize confrontation, argumentation, and labeling; 'roll' with resistance; and facilitate optimism and self-efficacy. This non-directive, supportive, reflective therapist style has been found to generate less resistance from clients, to be more successful in engaging them in the therapeutic process, and to predict better outcomes than a more directive, confrontive style (Miller et al., 1993).

Twelve Step Facilitation

There were a number of reasons to include an intervention based on the Twelve Step principles of AA. These programs are available in communities throughout the world. For many people, AA is the only resource ever used to resolve a drinking problem (Hasin & Grant, 1995). Many rehabilitation programs include AA meetings on-site and encourage their clients to become involved in community-based AA activities. The Twelve Step philosophy has had a strong influence on the evolution of alcohol rehabilitation programs such as the Minnesota Model, which relies heavily on AA principles (e.g., Cook, 1988; Spicer, 1993; McElrath, 1997). Although there are few well-controlled studies supporting the clinical effectiveness of AA (e.g., Tonigan et al., 1996b), there is documentation of a generally positive relationship between drinking outcome and attendance at AA meetings or involvement in AA activities such as having a sponsor, doing 'Big Book' and other readings, and working the Twelve Steps (e.g., Emrick, 1987; Montgomery et al., 1995; Timko et al., 1995; Morgenstern et al., 1997; Watson et al., 1997). Additionally, involvement in AA may also decrease healthcare utilization and related costs (Humphreys & Moos, 1996). Research on characteristics of AA affiliates suggested that matching of clients with AA would be important to investigate (Tonigan & Hiller-Sturmhofel, 1994; Galaif & Sussman, 1995; Humphreys, 1997). However, AA and other Twelve Step programs have high levels of attrition, which suggests that many people do not receive the maximum benefit from AA involvement (e.g., Godlaski et al., 1997). Because of this, the Project MATCH Twelve Step Facilitation (TSF) therapy focused on facilitating active and continued involvement in Twelve Step activities, rather than on the content of the Twelve Steps.

The TSF intervention (Nowinski et al., 1992) emphasized attendance at AA meetings and active involvement in the AA program as a primary means of recovery. In addition, this intervention had a number of objectives related to the first three steps of AA. First, TSF was intended to facilitate 'acceptance,' which includes the realization that alcoholism is a chronic progressive disease, that life has become unmanageable because of alcohol, that willpower is insufficient to overcome the problem, and that abstinence is the only alternative. Second, TSF was designed to facilitate the individual's 'surrender,' which involves giving oneself over to a higher power, accepting the fellowship of other recovering alcoholics, and following the recovery activities laid out by the Twelve Step program. Further, the TSF therapy process attempted to instill hope for recovery. Clients were given an opportunity to examine their thinking patterns (e.g., rationalization, denial), emotions, behaviors, interpersonal relationships, social activities, and spirituality. They were asked to consider how each is related to drinking and how changes in each area would enhance their chances of sobriety. In addition to helping the individual incorporate the AA belief system, TSF encouraged the person to turn to AA to gain support in changing habits that maintain drinking, and to increase social involvement with other AA members.

TSF was delivered in 12 sessions over the course of 12 weeks. A series of core therapy sessions, standard for all clients, addressed the major therapeutic goals described above. Several elective sessions were more individualized and could be used flexibly by the therapist. Topics included genograms (an inventory of relatives used to demonstrate that alcoholism is a disease that runs in families), enabling (behaviors of others that have facilitated the individual's continued drinking), people–places–routines (an examination of the contexts of drinking that are considered important to change), emotions (hunger, anger, loneliness, fatigue), moral inventories (a review of some of the 'wrongs' done while drinking and related guilt that might threaten recovery), interpersonal relationships, and lifestyle.

Each session also provided supplemental 'recovery tasks' such as AA-related homework assignments and Twelve Step readings to be done between sessions. Clients were encouraged to keep a diary, which was reviewed at the beginning of each session, in which they kept track of their reactions to AA meetings, explored why meetings were not attended, and recorded reactions to assigned readings and other recovery tasks. They were also asked to monitor when, where, and with whom they experienced urges to drink or actual slips, how they handled these, and what they could do in the future (e.g., going to a meeting, going to an AA social activity, calling their sponsor). Finally, two conjoint sessions with a significant other, focusing on the specific topics of enabling and detachment in relationships, were possible as part of the 12 sessions.

Within this context, the therapist educated the client about AA, its view of alcoholism, the Twelve Steps, the importance of the fellowship of AA, and the role of the sponsor. The therapist also used the client's reports of experiences between sessions to facilitate involvement in AA activities. The TSF approach involved a fairly active role on the part of the therapist. Although it was not necessary for TSF therapists to be in recovery themselves, such a status was thought to facilitate their role as an advocate for AA involvement.

A common misconception is that TSF is the *same* as AA. While they are clearly related, they are not equivalent. In contrast to the group-centered approach of AA, TSF is a form of individual psychotherapy delivered in accordance with written guidelines by a professional therapist or counselor.

Internal versus external validity

An important strength of Project MATCH was its methodological rigor, assuring a high level of internal validity. Considerable effort was made to maintain the integrity of the therapies through the development and use of treatment manuals, therapist hiring guidelines, and centralized training and supervision. However, many of the decisions made in the interest of conducting a highly controlled clinical trial, while clearly advantageous in research terms, may reduce external validity or generalizability.

One decision that required a compromise between methodological considerations and clinical practice was the choice to employ an individual therapy format. Group therapy is the most common form of treatment for substance abusers, having surpassed individual therapy as the psychotherapeutic intervention of choice (Stinchfield et al., 1994). Group therapy is also relatively cost effective, because therapists can treat more clients in the same amount of time. While group therapy has a high degree of clinical relevance and practical utility in the treatment community, four disadvantages are associated with this approach in the context of a clinical trial:

1. there is greater difficulty in standardizing group protocols, training guidelines, and implementation of treatments;

2. groups are often conducted with co-therapists, adding another factor to the analysis;
3. groups are likely to produce cohort effects, raising a question about the appropriate unit of analysis – the group as a whole, or individual clients within the group;
4. it is more difficult to investigate the nature of client–treatment or client–therapist interactions in group than in individual approaches.

A second example of a compromise between internal and external validity involves the efforts to purify each of the three treatments. Although relatively pure therapies are necessary in psychotherapy research to allow the active ingredients of the interventions to be identified and evaluated, pure therapies are difficult to find in most clinical practice settings. It is not uncommon for therapists to integrate aspects of different therapeutic approaches. For example, a CBT therapist, in addition to using interventions commonly associated with this approach, is likely to use strategies aimed at enhancing motivation and commitment to change, and to encourage active involvement in a Twelve Step program to sustain abstinence beyond the time limits of formal treatment.

Implementation of the therapies

Development of treatment manuals

Each of the three Project MATCH therapies was described in a detailed therapist manual. Treatment manuals facilitate the training of therapists; provide specific, identifiable, and replicable treatment procedures; and serve as a basis for developing measurement systems to objectively compare therapies and assess therapist conformity within an intended approach (Luborsky & DeRubeis, 1984; Carroll et al., 1994). Treatment manuals also serve to reduce 'noise' in psychotherapy efficacy trials by decreasing the variability in outcome due to therapist effects (Crits-Christoph et al., 1991).

The TSF and MET manuals were created as entirely new products based on descriptions in the literature, clinical reports, and the experience of the investigators. The CBT manual was based largely on a pre-existing manual (Monti et al., 1989), with substantial additions and modifications made for Project MATCH. Emphasis was placed on minimizing overlap across the three therapies.

Whereas it was fairly straightforward to specify the components of the cognitive–behavioral approach and to incorporate them into the therapist manual, it was much more difficult to specify TSF. To assure that TSF would typify the counseling found in Twelve Step-oriented treatment programs that seek to foster enduring relationships with AA, senior staff were consulted at the Hazelden Foundation, a leading proponent of the Twelve Step approach. They felt that the final TSF manual accurately reflected Twelve Step counseling approaches.

Each Project MATCH treatment manual consists of an overview of the intervention and its goals, general instructions regarding use of the manual, a description of the structure of the treatment sessions, and guidelines for dealing with potential client problems (e.g., outside crises, missed sessions, resistance) in ways that are consistent with the treatment approach. For Outpatient clients, guidelines focused on achieving abstinence and managing early recovery; for Aftercare clients, emphasis was placed on the prevention of relapse and the maintenance of sobriety. Additionally, detailed instructions were provided for each treatment session.

Selection of therapists

Individuals serving as therapists in Project MATCH went through an extensive selection and training process. To achieve consistency of intervention delivery across Clinical Research Units (CRUs) and treatment conditions, therapists were required to meet the following selection criteria:

- completion of a master's degree in counseling, psychology, social work, or a closely related field, or certification as an alcoholism counselor;
- at least 2 years of clinical experience after completion of degree or certification;
- submission of a taped clinical work sample to the CRU Principal Investigator and to the Coordinating Center for review;
- commitment to, and experience with, the Project MATCH treatment that the therapist would be conducting;
- experience treating alcoholics or a closely related clinical population.

Therapists were nested within the three treatment conditions; that is, each therapist conducted only one type of intervention. In contrast to a design in which therapists deliver all treatments, this approach had both methodological and clinical advantages. Methodologically, it minimized the likelihood that therapists would have different levels of experience and skill across the three therapies. It also reduced the potential for 'therapist drift,' exemplified by the use of techniques from treatments other than the target intervention. Drift from protocol guidelines not only threatens the integrity of the treatments, but also is more likely to occur at the extreme ends of the severity continuum where matching effects are expected to be strongest. When presented with challenging clinical problems, therapists would be more likely to draw from their clinical experience and manage clients in a manner consistent with manual guidelines.

The therapist selection criteria were designed to favor therapists representative of the usual practitioners of the study treatments and at the same time achieve comparability of therapists across treatments. For example, CBT therapists were usually psychologists with advanced degrees who had experience treating alcoholics. As TSF required familiarity with and commitment to AA principles, therapists selected for this treatment condition were predominantly individuals who had gone through Twelve Step recovery themselves, had been abstinent for several years, and were certified alcoholism counselors. Finally, because MET was a relatively new therapy, and there was no pool of available therapists with previous experience in MET, therapists were selected who typically had experience in either client-centered or family therapy. Comparison of the therapists across the three conditions confirmed the anticipated pattern of differences on alcohol use and recovery measures, but few differences were found with respect to personality attributes (Project MATCH Research Group, 1998d).

Therapist training

Another strategy designed to reduce variability across therapists at different sites was centralized training and supervision. Using methods developed in previous large-scale collaborative studies (Weissman et al., 1982; Elkin et al., 1985), all therapists attended an intensive training seminar that systematically reviewed the rationale for Project MATCH, the treatment manual for the specific intervention the therapist would be delivering, and taped examples of treatment sessions. Also included in the training were role-play exercises and extensive discussion of challenges related to treating a heterogeneous client population while following manual guidelines. Each therapist was then assigned a minimum of two training cases, which were conducted according to the protocol for their assigned treatment.

All training case sessions were videotaped and sent to the Coordinating Center (CC) for a review of:

- adherence to manual guidelines;
- level of skillfulness in treatment delivery;
- maintenance of appropriate structure and focus;
- empathy and facilitation of the therapeutic alliance;
- nonverbal behavior.

CC supervisors, who were highly experienced proponents of the treatments they supervised, reviewed all training sessions and provided weekly individual supervision to each therapist via telephone. Supplemental on-site supervision was provided weekly by the Project Coordinator at each CRU.

Therapists were certified by the CC supervisors following successful completion of training cases. Therapists whose performance on initial cases was inadequate were assigned additional training cases. Across conditions, therapists completed an average of 26 supervised training sessions before certification. Five therapist candidates were not certified, primarily because they had mixed therapeutic orientations which they could not adequately purify.

Ongoing supervision of therapists

Following the training and certification phase, supervision shifted to quality control. To maintain consistent quality of treatment delivery across sites and to prevent therapist drift during the main phase of the study, all sessions were videotaped and one-third of each client's sessions were reviewed by the supervisors. Telephone supervision was provided monthly by the CC supervisors and supplemented with weekly on-site supervision at each CRU.

All monitored treatment sessions were rated for therapist skillfulness, adherence to manual guidelines, and delivery of manual-specified active ingredients unique to each approach. These ratings were sent monthly to the project coordinators at each site to alert local supervisors of therapist drift. Therapists whose performance deviated in either quality or adherence to the manual were 'redlined' by the CC supervisors, and the frequency of supervision was increased until performance returned to acceptable levels.

Treatment compliance

Overall, clients in the three treatments completed approximately 67% of the recommended treatment sessions, a higher rate than is usually found in alcoholism treatment outcome studies (Mattson et al., 1998). On average, CBT clients attended more sessions ($M = 8.3$, SD $= 4.2$) than participants in TSF ($M = 7.4$, SD $= 4.3$) or MET ($M = 3.2$, SD $= 1.3$). Conversely, those in MET completed a higher proportion of sessions ($M = 0.80$, SD $= 0.32$) than those in CBT ($M = 0.68$, SD $= 0.35$) or TSF ($M = 0.63$, SD $= 0.36$). However, the former were requested to attend fewer sessions (four) than their counterparts in the other two conditions (12). Although statistically significant, these differences were not considered clinically meaningful (Project MATCH Research Group, 1997a; Mattson et al., 1998).

Discriminability of the therapies

Treatment manuals provide a basis for assuring the integrity of treatment over the course of its delivery and for assessing whether one treatment is discriminable from other approaches. Considerable effort was made to identify the 'active ingredients' or mechanisms of action of each therapy to minimize overlap and to heighten the distinctiveness of the treatments. Table 4.1 presents a comparison of the three therapies across a number of conceptual, therapeutic, and logistical dimensions.

Empirical data suggest that the procedures used to minimize overlap across the therapies were successful (Carroll et al., 1998). The Tape Rating Scale (TRS), consisting of a series of Likert-type items and a rating manual, was developed to evaluate the extent to which the therapies as delivered included the purported active ingredients specific to each inter-vention, while minimizing the active ingredients of the other two therapies (see Carroll et al., 1998, for details regarding scale development, rater reliability, and internal consistency). After completing a training and certification protocol, 19 experienced clinicians (who were not Project MATCH therapists) used the TRS to rate videotapes of 1716 therapy sessions. The three therapies were rated as distinct and discriminable; that is, study therapists were rated as making frequent use of techniques associated with their respective treatment manuals and relatively little use of techniques associated with the other two approaches. Further analyses indicated that these differences were attributable to the type of treatment, rather than to the rater, the therapist, the clinical site, or a site by treatment interaction (see Carroll et al., 1998).

Another potential source of overlap of specific ingredients in Project MATCH was AA attendance by clients. Because encouragement of AA attendance and reinforcement of Twelve Step work were the principal active ingredients of TSF, maintaining the purity of the treatments would have required that AA involvement not be part of the other two treatments. However, prohibiting participants from attending AA meetings would be unfeasible and possibly unethical, and some clients would attend meetings no matter what they were told. It was therefore decided to assume a neutral posture on this issue in the CBT and MET therapies (where therapists neither encouraged nor discouraged AA attendance) and to monitor participants' AA attendance as a process variable. As expected, clients in the TSF condition attended more AA meetings than did those in either CBT or MET (Carroll et al., 1998). Thus, the efforts to develop distinctive therapies appear to have been successful.

Unique versus nonspecific treatment components

Despite efforts to maintain the distinctiveness of study treatments, a host of nonspecific elements across treatments may contribute to treatment outcome. These include establishing rapport, providing support, empathic responding, setting limits, offering education, and furnishing a convincing therapeutic rationale (Kazdin, 1979). If matching effects are to be found, they will depend on the presence of unique treatment elements operating against a background of potentially powerful, nonspecific elements common to all of the treatments. Conversely, the presence of strong, nonspecific elements could be responsible for the absence of matching.

Considerable effort was made to distinguish between the unique active ingredients of each treatment (i.e., the theoretical mechanisms of action) which should *not* overlap, and nonspecific elements common to all treatments, which would be likely to overlap and therefore should be comparable across treatments. For example, emphasis on the identification of cognitions related to drinking and the development of specific coping skills should be present only in CBT. Similarly, therapist prescriptions for attending AA meetings and invoking a Higher Power should be present only in TSF. In contrast, elements such as the therapeutic alliance and therapist skillfulness should be as similar as possible across conditions to avoid a potential source of confounding between treatments.

Analyses examining nonspecific aspects of treatment indicated that, in general, the three therapies did not differ with respect to these dimensions (Carroll et al., 1998). The level of therapist skillfulness (as defined by ratings of general clinical skill, therapist empathy, and therapist nonverbal behavior) and the clients' perception of the working alliance between client

Table 4.1. *Contrasts among Project MATCH therapies*[a]

Therapeutic dimension	Twelve Step Facilitation	Cognitive–behavioral therapy	Motivational therapy
Goals of treatment	Accept alcoholism and understand it as a progressive, fatal disease Facilitate involvement in AA	Master coping behaviors as effective alternatives to alcohol use Increase self-efficacy	Maximize motivation and commitment to change drinking Increase self-efficacy
Therapy approach	Disease oriented	Cognitive–behavioral	Motivational
Agent of change	Fellowship/higher power	Mastery of skills	Client
Labeling	Labeling the client as 'alcoholic' is encouraged, as this label provides the framework for treatment Acceptance of the diagnosis is necessary	Labeling discouraged; alcohol abuse/dependence is conceived as learned behavior that can be broken down into a finite set of discrete problem situations and behaviors	Labeling is strongly discouraged
Control	Emphasis on loss of control. The client has the disease of alcoholism, and is powerless to control drinking. Clients can control whether they have the next drink and whether they use AA	Emphasis on self-control. Client can learn to understand and better control the decision-making process. Client can exert self-control by choosing alternative behaviors and cognitions	Emphasis on choice. Client has full control over the decision to alter drinking
Responsibility	Client not responsible for disease of alcoholism but is responsible for own sobriety by 'working' the Twelve Step program	Client responsible for own behavior. Emphasis on enhancing self-efficacy through skills training	Client responsible for own choices. Emphasis on autonomy
Strategies for addressing ambivalence and motivation	Remember last drunk. Alcoholism is a disease that motivates denial. Educate client about 'sinister' aspects of the disease. Current problems attributed to disease	Review positive/negative consequences of decisions to drink or stay abstinent. Instill belief that effective coping will provide alternatives to drinking	Acknowledge validity of client's feelings. Provide feedback. Empathic listening with double-sided reflection. Primacy of client's choice. Deploy discrepancy. Elicit self-motivational statements

	'Do not think you can control the consequences of use'	'You can learn skills to avoid lapses'	'It's up to you whether you drink or not'
Importance of abstinence	Total abstinence recommended, nonabstinent drinking goal strongly discouraged	Total abstinence recommended, nonabstinent drinking goal accepted	Total abstinence recommended, nonabstinent drinking goal accepted
Coping behaviors	AA fellowship and network provide a ready-made set of strategies	Individualized strategies, generalizable problem-solving approach. Specific training in drink-refusal skills, urge control, altering cognitions, emergency planning, social skills, affect management, and job-seeking skills	Development of coping strategies encouraged, but these are *not provided* by the therapist. Client encouraged to use personally effective coping strategies
Negative cognitions	Generally interpreted as evidence of rationalization and denial (e.g., 'stinking thinking')	Identified, examined, and challenged; encourage alternative perceptions/cognitions	Accepted as valid; met with exploration, reflection, and feedback
Phone calls/crises	Refer client to AA/sponsor. 'Use the fellowship' Two permissible emergency sessions	Encourage client to implement coping strategies Two permissible emergency sessions	Meet client's concerns with reflection and elicitation of client's plan of action Two permissible emergency sessions

[a]Adapted and reprinted with permission from Donovan et al. (1994) *Journal of Studies on Alcohol*, Supplement No. 12, 138–48. Copyright by Alcohol Research Documentation, Inc., Rutgers Center of Alcohol Studies, Piscataway, NJ 08855.

and therapist were comparable across the three treatments. It is of note that greater perceived working alliance was found to be predictive in the Outpatient arm of better treatment outcome, even after the effects attributable to the type of treatment were taken into account (Connors et al., 1997).

Clinical deterioration guidelines

Although there is a strong desire in any treatment study to have participants complete their assigned intervention, some clients may not improve, and others may even worsen to a point where it is unsafe to continue treatment. This is even more likely in treatment matching research that includes clients who, in addition to the usual vulnerability to physical, psychological, or alcohol-related problems during the course of the study interventions, may be 'mismatched' to treatment.

Two approaches were taken to deal with this potential problem. First, therapists were permitted to offer clients up to two emergency sessions to help them manage clinical crises. Emergency sessions were conducted using techniques consistent with each treatment type. When a crisis arose, CBT therapists modeled a problem-solving approach, TSF therapists encouraged their clients to deepen their involvement in AA, and MET therapists invited their clients to explore the resources already available to them. A total of 64 emergency sessions were conducted across the three therapies and two arms of the trial, a relatively small number considering the trial's large sample size ($n = 1726$).

If the emergency sessions were insufficient and the client continued to deteriorate, study staff had to decide whether to remove the client from the treatment protocol. To maintain a high standard of both clinical care and treatment integrity across therapies and CRUs, trial-wide criteria were adopted for determination of clinical deterioration and removal from the clinical arm of the trial. These included the onset of: (1) significant suicidal or homicidal ideations or attempts; (2) acute psychosis; (3) severe cognitive or physical impairment; or (4) extensive drinking or drug use that could not be managed on an outpatient basis. Clients removed from the treatment portion of the trial remained in the research sample and were assessed at follow-up evaluations and included in statistical analyses.

To promote uniform application of clinical deterioration criteria across sites, a Clinical Care Committee was formed to review cases and provide guidance when it was unclear whether clients should be referred to a more intensive intervention. A total of 57 clients were withdrawn from treatment due to clinical deterioration. Although more cases were withdrawn from the Outpatient ($n = 30$) than from the Aftercare ($n = 27$) study, the rates were roughly proportional to the numbers of participants enrolled in each arm (Outpatient, 3.1%; Aftercare, 3.4%). MET accounted for almost half (40%) of all cases of deterioration, followed by CBT (30%) and TSF (30%). Continued or excessive drinking was the most commonly cited reason for withdrawal (46 cases) and was involved in 80% of cases of clinical deterioration.

A total of 27 participants died over the course of the trial (three during the treatment phase; 24 during the follow-up period), representing 1.6% of the client sample. Over three-quarters (76.9%) of the deaths occurred among Aftercare clients. The most common cause of death was medical problems. Although alcohol seems to have contributed in some way to the death of 12 clients, the role of alcohol in the majority of cases was unknown. Clinical deterioration cases and death reports were forwarded to the Data Monitoring Board, the group charged with safety and ethical oversight of the trial (see Chapter 2).

Costs of Project MATCH therapies

A practical question that has obvious policy relevance is the cost that would be involved in implementing Project MATCH therapies in community treatment settings. Cost estimates derived from the clinical research settings in which the trial was conducted would surely generate overestimates, given the intensity of therapist training and supervision provided. Cisler and colleagues (1998) estimated the costs of the therapies as actually delivered at three Project MATCH CRUs, as well as the likely costs of replicating them in community treatment settings. The estimates of the direct clinical costs per client were based on four primary cost components.

The first component was the average number of contact hours within each therapy, based on the percent of completed sessions. On average, CBT clients had 8.14 contact hours (67% of scheduled sessions completed), MET clients had 3.19 hours (75% of scheduled sessions), and the TSF clients had 7.40 contact hours (67% of scheduled sessions). The second cost estimate was based on the recommended minimal therapist professional qualifications and the corresponding hourly wages (costs per therapist per client hour). The third component of the cost estimates was the expense associated with intake assessments needed to conduct the therapies as presented in the treatment manuals. The MET feedback session required a fairly lengthy part of the intake assessment, averaging 3 hours. In contrast, no specialized assessments were considered necessary to conduct either CBT or TSF. The final direct cost component involved treatment materials, such as copies of the 'Big Book' (Alcoholics Anonymous, 1976), *Living Sober* (Alcoholics Anonymous, 1975), and other materials used in TSF.

In addition to these direct client costs, two other costs were considered. The first was the institutional indirect costs, which refer to the general support services required in a clinical setting. These were estimated at 30% of direct costs. The second factor was initial therapist training and ongoing supervision.

Based on these assumptions and cost projections, three sets of estimates were derived for the replication of the Project MATCH therapies in community treatment settings:

1. the direct clinical cost per client;
2. the training and supervision costs;
3. the total costs per client.

Figure 4.1 compares the three therapies in terms of the three types of cost. With respect to the direct costs, MET averaged $276 per client (range across sites, $180–$394), TSF averaged $313 per client ($144–$577), and CBT averaged $333 per client ($140–$606). The total cost per client, which adds 30% institutional indirect costs on to these estimates, was $359 ($234–$512) for MET; $407 ($187–$750) for TSF; and $433 ($182–$788) for CBT. Finally, the average per therapist costs for initial training and supervision were $1762 ($1334–$2620) for MET; $2278 ($1511–$3229) for TSF; and $2404 ($1514–$3461) for CBT. Based on these estimates, the costs for training and supervising one therapist to provide an average dosage of a given therapy to one client within an institutional setting were estimated as follows: MET, $2397; TSF, $2685; and CBT, $2837.

According to Cisler et al. (1998), Project MATCH treatments appear to be at the higher end of the spectrum of cost estimates in community settings (Holder et al., 1991), perhaps because a large proportion of community-based programs provide less expensive group therapy. Nevertheless, the costs of delivering the Project MATCH treatments need to be weighed against their potential effectiveness in treating alcohol problems (see Chapters 7, 8, and 9). Finally, the cost analyses indicate that the

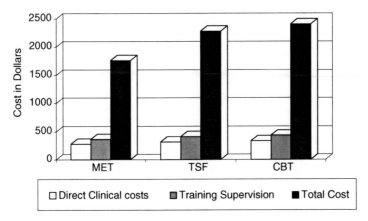

Figure 4.1 Estimates (in US$) of direct clinical costs, training and supervision costs, and total costs per client to deliver Motivational Enhancement Therapy (MET), Twelve Step Facilitation (TSF) therapy and Cognitive–Behavioral Therapy (CBT).

differences among the three treatment modalities are less than might be anticipated, to the extent that the four-session MET was only marginally less expensive than the two 12-session treatments. The apparent cost advantage of MET relative to CBT and TSF was diminished by the costs of assessment feedback, which were not present in the other therapies, and the fact that MET clients attended proportionately more sessions.

Summary and conclusions

Lindström (1992) and others have noted that, in order to find matching effects, it is necessary to have therapies that are clearly differentiated, well defined, and for which there is careful specification of active ingredients unique to each treatment being compared. The therapy selection, development, and implementation process used in Project MATCH produced three therapies that met these criteria. The therapies were shown to be unique, discriminable, and capable of producing a strong working alliance between clients and therapists. Moreover, more than 80 therapists were trained and supervised to deliver these therapies with a high degree of fidelity. Finally, the costs of delivering these individual therapies in community settings, although more expensive than typical outpatient treatment, were nevertheless reasonable given their quality and potential effectiveness.

5

Client characteristics and implementation of the research protocol

ALLEN ZWEBEN, FRANCES K. DEL BOCA, MARGARET E. MATTSON, AND BONNIE MCREE

Implementation means putting a plan into action. Project MATCH required the recruitment of a large and diverse group of alcohol-dependent research participants, and these clients are described in this chapter. As expected, clients recruited for the Outpatient arm demonstrated less severe alcohol-related problems than clients recruited into the Aftercare arm from residential or day-hospital treatment programs. With some exceptions, participants were found to be broadly representative of client populations in alcoholism treatment. Also discussed are the crucial implementation measures that determine the internal validity of a clinical trial: centralized random assignment procedures, quality control measures, checks on measurement reliability, and research compliance procedures. Data are presented to indicate that these procedures were successful in minimizing threats to internal and external validity.

The implementation of a multisite treatment matching trial is a complex and challenging task. As indicated in Chapter 2, the Coordinating Center (CC) sought to maintain the independence of the treatment and research components of the trial by concentrating each function in a separate location under the supervision of different investigators. The present chapter focuses on the implementation of the research protocol, specifically the recruitment of appropriate research participants for the trial; the random assignment of clients to treatment conditions; the training and supervision of staff at diverse clinical sites to assure adherence to a standard set of procedures for data collection; the facilitation of client participation in the research protocol; the collection of data that were complete, timely, and accurate; and the processing and management of data from multiple research sites. This chapter also presents data to underscore the utility of these methods.

Participant enrollment

Client characteristics

Three aims were pursued in recruiting clients for Project MATCH. The first was to generate large and diverse participant samples suitable for testing a broad range of treatment matching hypotheses in the two arms of the trial (Zweben et al., 1994). A second objective concerned generalizability. Recognizing that the requirements of a clinical trial inevitably restrict the range of participants enrolled, efforts were made to ensure that participants were as broadly representative as possible of the client populations found in alcoholism treatment settings. A final aim was to recruit women and ethnic minorities, who have often been under-represented in treatment research, in sufficient numbers to test the effects of gender and ethnicity on treatment outcomes.

A wide variety of strategies was used to recruit participants. In the Outpatient arm, advertisements were placed in newspapers and in the broadcast media. Research staff distributed brochures, conducted workshops, and employed other methods to inform relevant agencies about the project. In the Aftercare arm, formal affiliations were developed between the Clinical Research Units (CRUs) and specialized inpatient or residential alcoholism treatment facilities (e.g., private hospitals, Veterans Administration facilities, state-funded programs), where on-site representatives were often employed to facilitate the flow of referrals into the study. These strategies enabled the CRUs to meet sample size requirements within the 2-year time period allotted for recruitment. The initial goal was 800 participants for each of the study arms, or a total of 1600. The final sample sizes were 952 clients in the Outpatient arm and 774 participants (representing 27 different inpatient programs) in the Aftercare study, for a total of 1726 participants.

Table 5.1 describes the Outpatient and Aftercare samples. Participants were diverse in terms of demographic variables such as gender, ethnicity, relationship status, and current employment. Recruitment objectives for women and minorities were met. Across the two study arms, 25% of clients were women, and 20% were members of minority groups. Although virtually all participants – 95% of Outpatients, 98% of Aftercare clients – met criteria for alcohol dependence as assessed by the Structured Clinical Interview for DSM-III-R (Spitzer & Williams, 1985), Table 5.1 indicates that there was considerable variation in terms of alcohol involvement and other problems.

Table 5.1. *Characteristics of Outpatient and Aftercare clients*

Variable	Outpatient (*n* = 952)	Aftercare (*n* = 774)
Gender (%)		
Male	72	80
Female	28	20
Age (mean, SD)	38.9 (10.7)	41.9 (11.1)
Ethnicity (%)		
White	80	80
African American	6	15
Hispanic	12	3
Other	2	1
Years of formal education (mean, SD)	13.4 (2.2)	13.1 (2.1)
Relationship status (%)		
Couple	36	34
Single	64	66
Employment status (%)		
Employed	51	48
Not employed	49	52
Prior alcohol treatment (%)		
Yes	45	62
No	55	38
Number of alcohol-dependence symptoms (mean, SD)[a]	5.8 (1.9)	6.8 (1.9)
Alcohol consumption[b]		
Percent Days Abstinent (mean, SD)	34 (30)	27 (30)
Drinks per Drinking Day (mean, SD)	13.5 (8.0)	20.5 (12.1)
Drinker Inventory of Consequences (mean, SD)[b,c]	45.8 (21.6)	59.5 (23.2)
Illicit drug use[b] (%)		
Yes	44	32
No	56	68
Beck Depression Inventory (mean, SD)	9.8 (8.0)	10.6 (8.6)
ASI Psychiatric Severity[d] (mean, SD)	0.19 (0.19)	0.23 (0.21)
ASI criminal behavior (%)		
Alcohol-related crimes	61	67
Other crimes	39	40

[a]Measured by the Structured Clinical Interview for DSM-IV (SCID) for the 90-day period prior to enrollment; symptom counts range from 1 to 9.
[b]Assessed for a 90-day period prior to enrollment.
[c]Total scale score.
[d]Composite score derived from the Addiction Severity Index; higher scores indicate higher levels of severity.

As expected, Outpatient and Aftercare clients differed in ways consistent with the functions of outpatient and residential treatment (Goodman et al., 1992; Timko et al., 1993; Monahan & Finney, 1996). Participants in the Outpatient arm tended to be younger, more residentially stable, and less dependent on alcohol than those in the Aftercare study. As shown in Table 5.1, Outpatient clients drank more frequently (73% of the 90 days prior to enrollment, compared to 66%) and more intensively (20.5 Drinks per Drinking Day, compared to 13.5) than their Aftercare counterparts. Prior alcoholism treatment was more often reported among those in Aftercare (62%) than among those in the Outpatient study (45%). Although individuals currently dependent on other drugs (except for marijuana) were excluded, a sizable minority of participants reported illicit drug use (44% Outpatient, 32% Aftercare). However, the use of other drugs was relatively infrequent. For example, the median frequency of marijuana use ranged from 1 day during the 90-day pre-treatment period for Aftercare women to 4 days for Outpatient men. Lifetime Axis I (non-substance use disorder) diagnoses were found in 52% and 59% of Outpatient and Aftercare clients, respectively, and a high proportion reported alcohol-related (61% and 67%) as well as other (39% and 40%) crimes.

To enhance generalizability, coerced treatment referrals (e.g., Driving Under the Influence offenders and individuals on probation or parole) were accepted if their legal restrictions did not preclude them from random assignment to one of the three Project MATCH treatments. In the Aftercare study, the average length of stay in an inpatient or day treatment program was consistent with the prevailing policies of health maintenance organizations or insurance carriers for the treatment of alcohol-related problems, ranging from 7 to 44 days in treatment, with a mean of 20.9 days.

Examination of the characteristics of excluded and selected participants suggests that recruitment procedures succeeded in identifying a broad range of clients who were similar to those seen in Outpatient and residential treatment settings. A review of screening data for 4481 potential participants showed that 459 (10%) refused to take part in the trial; most cited logistical reasons, including transportation problems (45%), lack of available time (21%), and plans to relocate (17%). Of the remaining 4022 potential participants, 2296 (57%) were found to be ineligible for treatment (Project MATCH Research Group, 1997a).

Further support for the general representativeness of Project MATCH participants is provided by Velasquez et al. (2000), who compared clients enrolled in Project MATCH to those who were not enrolled at one Aftercare site where comprehensive screening was conducted at the primary recruitment facility. Those not enrolled in the trial were categorized as either ineligible for the study or eligible but declining to participate. As expected, differences were found between those eligible and those ineligible in terms of plans to move, available transportation, identification of a 'locator' to facilitate future contact, and distance from the clinic. The groups did not differ, however, on a variety of demographic and severity measures, including pre-treatment drinking levels, recent drug use, job and residential stability, past psychiatric history, aggressive behavior, suicidal tendencies, and legal problems. There were several significant, albeit small, differences in age, education, and ethnicity. Ineligible volunteers were somewhat older and less educated than the study participants. There was also a higher percentage of Caucasians in the ineligible group, compared with volunteers who were eligible but declined participation. Finally, clients who participated in the trial had significantly higher scores on the Alcohol Use Disorders Identification Test (AUDIT) than both of the other groups.

To summarize, all three recruitment objectives were met. First, large samples were recruited for the two arms of the trial, and the distribution of client characteristics within the study samples indicates considerable heterogeneity. Second, although inclusion/exclusion criteria clearly resulted in the absence of particular types of clients, and possibly those who were the most difficult to treat (most notably, those who were transient, psychotic or seriously drug dependent, or insufficiently motivated to complete inpatient or day-hospital treatment), comparison data from other samples suggest that participants were broadly representative of client populations found in alcoholism treatment settings. Perhaps most importantly, the level of alcohol problem severity (as evidenced by reported alcohol consumption, prior treatment experiences, and diagnostic symptoms), coupled with the prevalence of psychopathology and criminal behavior in the two samples, suggests that Project MATCH participants did not comprise a highly select group with a uniformly favorable treatment prognosis (Project MATCH Research Group, 1997a, 1997b). Third, women and ethnic minorities were well represented, permitting analyses of the effects of gender and minority group membership on treatment outcomes. Although gender was related to drinking outcomes (women fared better than men in the Aftercare arm; see Chapter 8), no differences were found for ethnicity.

Random assignment to treatment

The decision to conduct a randomized clinical trial (RCT) raised a methodological question about whether to randomize centrally at the CC or locally at the CRUs. Local randomization, although convenient, is potentially subject to deliberate or unintentional bias, but centralized allocation is difficult to implement in a way that provides timely initiation of treatment. The CC addressed this issue by developing a centralized procedure that provided timely allocations to experimental conditions with rapid communication regarding treatment assignment to the CRUs.

Although random assignment diminishes the potential for the confounding of participant characteristics with treatment assignment, it does not guarantee the even distribution of important client attributes across conditions. Rather than attempting to implement a stratification procedure to deal with this concern, a relatively untested but very promising approach, urn randomization, was adopted for use in the trial. This method adjusts the probabilities of assignment to different conditions as a function of the characteristics of participants already allocated to each treatment (Stout et al., 1994).

The allocation procedure included several steps designed to check the inclusion/exclusion criteria, generate a centralized client database, and perform the randomization function. CRU staff faxed a standardized form to the CC containing demographic data, as well as the specific information needed for the urn randomization program (e.g., participant gender, severity of alcohol dependence). Data were entered into the urn randomization computer program, which returned a treatment assignment and saved information in a participant database. CRUs were immediately notified of each assignment by a telephone call, which was also confirmed in writing via fax.

The centralized urn randomization procedure proved to be an important asset in conducting the trial. The potential for bias associated with a decentralized method was eliminated. When recruitment ended, client characteristics were, in fact, evenly balanced across cells in the study design (cf. Project MATCH Research Group, 1997a). The CC was able to maintain an up-to-date database of client characteristics and to generate accrual reports for each site and arm of the trial that were reviewed weekly by the Executive Committee. Sites that experienced difficulty with recruitment were identified and targeted for remediation in a timely fashion. Any trends with respect to shifts in client characteristics were also apparent.

Implementation of the research protocol

Training and supervision of research staff

The assessment battery, described in detail in Chapter 3, was implemented to ensure that accurate and comparable data were collected across the nine CRUs. The assessment protocol was complex in that a variety of methods was used, including personal interviews, self-administered questionnaires, computer-assisted diagnostic procedures, and cognitive performance tasks. In addition, the protocol required staff to contact collateral inform-ants and 'locators,' and to arrange for the collection, storage, and ship-ment of blood and urine specimens. Standardization of procedures was complicated by numerous factors, including differences in recruitment procedures, the length of the assessment battery (which required three sessions at baseline, in addition to preliminary screening), and the fre-quency of follow-up evaluations. Five interviews were conducted at 3-month intervals over the course of 15 months, and a sixth interview was conducted 39 months after treatment initiation in the Outpatient arm. Additionally, the duration of the project produced a moderate degree of staff turnover. Over the course of the trial, Project MATCH included 20 investigators, 95 therapy personnel (therapists and supervisors) and 157 project coordinators, research assistants, and ancillary staff.

Several mechanisms, some of which parallel those used to ensure that treatment was delivered consistently across sites (see Chapter 4), were used to address these standardization issues. These included: (1) the develop-ment of detailed instructional materials; (2) a centralized certification process for interviewers; (3) a common training experience for research staff at the multiple sites; and (4) ongoing monitoring and supervision to minimize 'drift.'

A detailed procedures manual was developed that outlined all of the research activities in the trial. This manual was updated as the trial progressed and new situations were encountered. Research personnel training was extensive. Research staff were brought to a common location for two multiple-day training seminars that included funding agency per-sonnel and presentations by the trial investigators. Training included the use of videotaped interviews to demonstrate proper interview techniques and the discussion of common questions and problem scenarios. A crucial component of the training experience was the opportunity to interview patients in a setting that permitted questions and group discussion.

Following the training seminars, the CC developed a certification protocol that required interviewers to submit videotaped practice interviews for review. In addition, a local training protocol was developed to facilitate the training of new staff and to assure periodic on-site review of interviews and procedures.

During the data collection phase of the trial, annual site visits were conducted at each CRU. These involved two or more representatives from the CC and, in some instances, a representative from the funding agency. All aspects of CRU functioning were examined, including organization, structure, communication, recruitment methods, confidentiality protection, client tracking, on-site training, local supervision, research and treatment compliance, adherence to the research protocol, interview administration, and data management (see McRee, 1998, for more details).

Reliability of measurement

A major concern in multisite trials is consistency of measurement across sites. This issue was particularly salient in Project MATCH because many of the key instruments were adapted or developed specifically for use in the trial, and several of these were administered via personal interviews. Several strategies were used to estimate and enhance reliability. First, although many instruments required some adaptation for use in the trial, one selection consideration was prior use of some version of the instrument with alcohol-dependent respondents. Second, because of the need for uniformity across sites, specific probes and coding instructions were added to relatively unstructured interviews such as the Structured Clinical Interview for DSM-IV (SCID). Third, within-site reliability was enhanced through the use of training exercises that could be conducted locally at the CRUs.

The primary mechanism for assessing reliability was a two-component study that evaluated the major instruments using a sample of research volunteers who were not Project MATCH participants (see Del Boca et al., 1994; Del Boca & Brown, 1996). For the cross-site component, staff were brought together at a common location and paired across CRUs to examine interrater reliability. A similar protocol was used to assess within-site reliability at the CRUs. To provide variability in relevant client characteristics, research participants for the two studies included both alcoholics in treatment and community volunteers.

Of particular interest were the specific variables derived from the major interview assessments in the trial. These included DSM-III-R diagnoses of alcohol-use disorders from the SCID; two primary matching variables, the Psychiatric Severity composite score from the Addiction Severity Index (ASI) and Support for Drinking measure from the Important People and Activities instrument; and the two major drinking outcome variables from the Form-90, Percent Days Abstinent and Drinks per Drinking Day. With the single exception of the ASI Psychiatric Severity score, all of these measures yielded high reliability coefficients, both across and within sites, for the two arms of the trial. Reliability estimates appeared to be attenuated for the ASI measure in part because a large number of respondents were asymptomatic.

In addition to the interview assessments, the test–retest reliability of several of the self-administered questionnaires was also examined. These included the Readiness to Change measure (Miller & Tonigan, 1996), the Ethanol Dependence Syndrome scale (Babor, 1996), the Alcoholics Anonymous Involvement scale (Tonigan et al., 1996a), measures of perceived social support (Rice & Longabaugh, 1996), and the Religious Background and Beliefs scale (Connors et al., 1996). Reliability was consistently high across measures.

Data processing and management

Data processing and management represent another aspect of the research enterprise where errors can threaten the validity of the findings. As with other research activities, these tasks could have been conducted locally or centrally. It was felt that local data input at the CRUs would be less error prone, and the CC developed data entry software that required double key entry verification at the sites. Data entry programs were designed to minimize errors (e.g., skip patterns were automated, valid value ranges were established). A training manual and detailed codebook were prepared. CRUs periodically transmitted the entered data to the CC, where an extensive data checking protocol was used to identify missing values, logical inconsistencies, and other anomalous entries, as well as to cross-check entered values with the CC client tracking database and other sources. The CC queried the CRUs regarding all questionable entries, and the CRUs, in turn, resolved each case. Data from the multiple sites were then aggregated by the CC and prepared for analysis.

An independent random audit of selected cases at each CRU was conducted prior to data analysis, and virtually all entries were found to be correct. The error rate, as assessed by discrepancies between responses on hard copy forms and entered data, was found to be far less than 1%. Thus, the procedures developed for data processing and management further reduced any random or systematic error that might have potentially threatened the validity of the results.

Participation in research activities

In addition to reliable assessment, the information gathered from research participants must be complete, timely, and accurate to avoid serious threats to the internal and external validity of the research design. Differential drop-out rates for treatment conditions threaten internal validity. Even if uniform across conditions, low rates of participation in follow-up evaluations compromise external validity if completers and drop-outs differ on variables potentially related to treatment success (e.g., alcohol problem severity). Because the research requirements in Project MATCH were particularly demanding, a number of strategies were used to enhance research participation. This section describes these strategies, along with data bearing on the success of these efforts (see Zweben et al., 1998, and Mattson et al., 1998, for more details).

Compliance enhancement strategies

Clear communication regarding roles and responsibilities

Recognizing that client and contextual factors contribute to non-compliance, the responsibility for ensuring that research requirements were met was shared by both staff and participants. Emphasis was placed on forging an alliance with the client to develop and maintain a commitment to the project. At the same time, research personnel worked to enhance participant compliance by clarifying requirements and creating a 'user-friendly' research environment. Thus, staff devoted considerable attention to orienting clients to the research participant role and explaining study procedures (e.g., scheduling of follow-up appointments, use of breathalyzer, roles and responsibilities of locators and collateral informants, collection of blood and urine specimens). Staff routinely reviewed these obligations over the course of the trial to maintain the client's active participation.

Minimizing logistical barriers

Clients in alcoholism treatment are often overwhelmed by problems with work, family, and personal finances. These problems may interfere with their active involvement in a clinical trial. Within the context of these circumstances, inconvenient office hours and poor transportation facilities can serve as major barriers to participation. Thus, efforts were made to create clinical research sites that were accessible to clients and responsive to their particular circumstances. Research sites were typically located on local bus routes, and bus tickets were routinely offered to individuals for whom the costs of transportation were a financial burden. Flexible appointment times were provided to accommodate the needs of clients whose employment or child-care situation might preclude them from attending assessment sessions. Some sites employed bilingual staff to facilitate the involvement of clients who had difficulty with English.

Compliance monitoring

Completion of study requirements was closely monitored by the CRUs and by the CC. The CC developed software for generating assessment session due dates and monitoring interview completions, including blood and urine collection and collateral informant contacts. The CRUs regularly transferred their local data to a centralized client-tracking database that was maintained at the CC. Reports regarding participation rates and data completeness were routinely reviewed by the trial's Executive Committee so that solutions to compliance problems could be formulated and implemented quickly.

Reminders and incentives

Compliance enhancement procedures included a variety of prompts, reinforcers, and incentives which were tailored to the needs of specific sites and individual clients. Sites were encouraged to send reminder letters and make telephone calls for assessment appointments, and participants who tended to reschedule appointments often were contacted well in advance of their interview due dates. Clients were consistently treated with courtesy, and they were verbally reinforced for completing research tasks. Some sites rewarded participants with Project MATCH favors such as mugs or tee-shirts. All clients received financial compensation for the completion of follow-up assessment sessions.

Special accommodations for 'hard-to-reach' clients

A small number of clients at every CRU consistently experienced difficulty in complying with research protocol demands. Basic compliance strategies (e.g., financial incentives and other reinforcers, reducing environmental barriers) were not sufficient to address the needs of these clients. While recognizing the ethical rights of these participants to refuse to perform research tasks, staff attempted to engage resistant clients in the project by accommodating their special needs. For example, individuals who were unable or unwilling to attend a follow-up session on site were given the option of home visits or telephone interviews (see Barrett & Morse, 1998).

Virtually all of the compliance enhancement strategies adopted in the trial were designed to communicate respect and concern for the clients' welfare. One potential consequence of this approach was the blurring of the distinction between the research and clinical functions in the trial. Thus, the performance of research personnel was carefully monitored to assure that they were centered on facilitating the cooperation of clients for purposes of obtaining accurate and complete data and not serving in an active helping role (i.e., addressing drinking and drinking-related problems).

Research compliance in Project MATCH

Indicators of Data Quality

To monitor research compliance, the CC client-tracking database was used to create aggregate and individual-level measures of data completeness and timeliness. Analyses of research compliance focused on fulfillment of study requirements during the trial's follow-up phase. Data accuracy was confirmed by comparing client self-reports of drinking with collateral informant reports and biological markers.

Data completeness

Aggregate rates of follow-up participation were calculated for each of the five assessment periods, in each of the two study arms. As shown in Table 5.2, follow-up interviews were conducted with 92% of Outpatient and 93% of Aftercare clients at the 15-month assessment point (1 year after the end of treatment), and blood samples were obtained for 82% and 83% of the

Table 5.2. *Rates and timeliness of data provision for each follow-up period*

	3 month	6 month	9 month	12 month	15 month	39 month
Outpatient arm						
Completed interviews (%)[a]	98	96	95	93	92	87
Blood samples (%)	90	—	85	—	82	73
Urine specimens (%)	92	—	85	—	85	—
Collateral nominations (%)[b]	86	—	84	—	81	80
Collateral interviews (%)	76	—	74	—	75	71
Days late for interview[c] (mean)	24.4	24.1	23.3	20.2	20.5	—
Aftercare arm						
Completed interviews (%)[a]	97	97	95	94	93	—
Blood samples (%)	86	—	84	—	83	—
Urine specimens (%)	88	—	84	—	85	—
Collateral nominations (%)[b]	90	—	89	—	85	—
Collateral interviews (%)	87	—	86	—	78	—
Days late for interview[c] (mean)	23.9	23.4	21.8	21.3	17.1	—

[a]Deceased clients are excluded from the computation of rates; completion rates include 'reconstructions,' i.e., instances where data were provided for the index period at a later follow-up time point.

[b]Nomination rates are based on the client's provision of information regarding a collateral informant, whereas interview rates indicate the proportion of clients for whom collateral interviews were actually completed. Clients were encouraged, but not required, to name collateral informants to corroborate verbal reports.

[c]Means are based only on completed interviews that took place following their due dates.

(From Mattson et al., 1998, p. 1333). Copyright 1998, Research Society on Alcoholism, Austin, TX. Adapted with permission.

participants, respectively. Collection rates for urine specimens at this time point were 85% for both arms of the trial. Collateral informant nominations were requested (but not required) and interviews (which necessitated the cooperation of the informant, as well as the client) were completed for 75% of Outpatient and 78% of Aftercare participants at the 15-month assessment point.

Completion rates were also calculated for the 3-year follow-up evaluation (39 months after treatment initiation) that was conducted with Outpatient clients. As shown in Table 5.2, 87% of the participants were interviewed, 73% provided blood samples (urine speciments were not collected), and collateral informant interviews were obtained for 71%.

Data timeliness

Follow-up evaluations were due at successive 90-day intervals starting from the date of the first treatment session. Timeliness of data collection was operationalized as the number of days past the due date that interviews were actually completed. As indicated in Table 5.2, timeliness was similar across the two study arms; participants were interviewed approximately 20 (Outpatient) and 17 (Aftercare) days past their 15-month session due dates.

Data accuracy

To evaluate data accuracy, the concordance across three data sources was examined – self-reported drinking, collateral informant reports, and standard biological indicators (four biochemical tests: serum gamma-glutamyl transpeptidase [GGTP], serum aspartate aminotransferase [ASAT], serum alanine aminotransferase [ALAT], and carbohydrate deficient transferrin [CDT]). The three types of measures were compared at the time of admission to treatment and 1 year after the end of treatment (Babor et al., 2000). Results comparing the three measures are presented Table 5.3.

Agreement between client self-reports and collateral reports was very high at treatment admission (97%); in contrast, liver function tests were relatively insensitive, with positive values for those who admitted drinking ranging from 29% for ASAT to 40% for GGTP. At the 15-month follow-up evaluation, the correspondence between client self-reports and collateral reports decreased to 85%, but agreement with blood chemistry values increased, ranging from 43% for ALAT to 52% for CDT. The discrepancies that did occur suggested that the self-report method was more

Table 5.3. *Correspondence among outcome measures: self-reports, collateral reports, and liver function tests*

Assessment point	Drinking measure comparison	Agreement (%)[a]	Under-reporting rate (%)[b]	Over-reporting rate (%)[c]
Baseline	Client/collateral informant (*n* = 1338)	97	<1	3
	Client/liver function tests			
	GGTP (*n* = 1580)	40	<1	60
	ASAT (*n* = 1580)	29	<1	71
	ALAT (*n* = 1580)	30	<1	70
One-year follow-up	Client/collateral informant (*n* = 1248)	85	4	12
	Client/liver function tests			
	GGTP (*n* = 1363)	52	4	44.4
	ASAT (*n* = 1363)	46	3	50.8
	ALAT (*n* = 1363)	43	4	53.7
	CDT (*n* = 1266)	57	5	39.1

[a]Agreement indicates the proportion of cases in which both sources of data were in agreement, that is, both indicated drinking, or both indicated abstinence.
[b]Under-reporting rate refers to situations wherein the client has denied drinking while the other source has indicated drinking.
[c]Over-reporting rate refers to situations wherein the client admits drinking but the other source indicated abstinence.
GGTP, serum gamma-glutamyl transpeptidase; ASAT, serum aspartate aminotransferase; ALAT, serum alanine aminotransferase; CDT, carbohydrate-deficient transferrin.
Adapted from Babor et al. (2000).

sensitive to the amount of drinking than were the biochemical measures. That is, most inconsistencies resulted from situations in which participants admitted in their verbal reports to drinking, but the concomitant collateral or biochemical data suggested abstinence (see Babor et al., 2000).

Correlates of research compliance

The aggregate indicators reviewed above indicate a high degree of data quality (completeness, timeliness, accuracy) and suggest that random and systematic measurement error had relatively little impact on the study's internal and external validity. This possibility was investigated further by examining correlates of follow-up session completion, an individual-level measure of research compliance. Twenty-five different variables covering a range of client factors (demographic characteristics; measures of alcohol involvement; psychological factors, such as motivation and depression; and personal circumstance indicators, such as social stability and insurance coverage) and treatment-related variables (e.g., CRU, treatment condition, recruitment method) were investigated. Relatively few variables emerged as significant predictors of research compliance. Measures of previous psychiatric treatment, sociopathy, and less rapid treatment initiation were associated with lower levels of follow-up completion. Differences in compliance were also related to CRU in both arms of the trial. Although statistically significant, the relationships tended to be small in magnitude, with no correlation exceeding a value of 0.15 (Mattson et al., 1998).

Participant characteristics were also examined in relation to the discrepancies among verbal reports of drinking, collateral reports, and biochemical markers (Babor et al., 2000). Compared with clients showing concordant results, those with discrepancies tended to have more severe drinking problems (e.g., more prior alcoholism treatments, higher levels of pretreatment drinking) and greater levels of cognitive impairment, factors which could potentially interfere with accurate recall. Overall, however, there were few significant associations between client attributes and drinking data discrepancies.

The association between compliance and treatment outcome

As discussed in Chapter 2, the Project MATCH research design did not include an untreated control group. Moreover, several decisions regarding procedures, although made in the interest of comprehensive assessment and compliance enhancement, had the potential to affect outcomes independent of the client's involvement in treatment. Assessment requirements were extensive, and measures focused on alcohol use and its consequences, which may have affected clients' concerns about their drinking or their motivations to reduce consumption levels. To promote research compliance, participants were made aware that the trial was a highly visible, national study, and they received considerable individualized attention.

High compliance rates, coupled with a dearth of information about the outcomes of clients lost to follow-up, made it difficult to assess the impact of factors relating to participation in the research protocol (e.g., frequent assessment) on treatment outcomes. One approach to understanding whether reductions in drinking were purely attributable to research participation was to examine the effects of differing levels of treatment compliance for those clients who had completed all research requirements. Clients were grouped into three treatment compliance groups (high, moderate, and low) based upon the proportion of therapy sessions completed. Repeated measures analysis of covariance (controlling for baseline drinking) was conducted for each of the primary drinking outcomes, using treatment compliance group and treatment condition – Cognitive–Behavioral Therapy (CBT), Motivational Enhancement Therapy (MET), and Twelve Step Facilitation (TSF) – as independent factors. The results of these analyses are presented in Table 5.4.

The treatment compliance group main effect was statistically significant in the analyses of both dependent variables. As shown in Table 5.4, clients in the high treatment compliance group consistently reported more favorable drinking outcomes than those in the low and moderate groups. Significant treatment compliance group by treatment condition interactions were also obtained for both outcome variables. Among high compliance participants, those in TSF had the most positive outcomes, with less marked effects in CBT and in MET (Mattson et al., 1998). Although the results were variable across the three treatments, level of participation in treatment was related to drinking outcomes for those participants who completed all research requirements (i.e., when level of research participation was controlled). This finding suggests that any reductions in drinking observed in Project MATCH cannot simply be attributed to the time and attention involved in assessment and other research activities. This analytic strategy cannot, of course, totally compensate for the absence of an assessment-only control group and does not eliminate the possibility that

Table 5.4. *Drinking outcomes by treatment compliance subgroups and treatment condition*

Treatment compliance	Percent Days Abstinent[a]			Drinks per Drinking Day[b]		
	Low ($n = 443$)	Moderate ($n = 224$)	High ($n = 884$)	Low ($n = 443$)	Moderate ($n = 224$)	High ($n = 884$)
CBT	0.70	0.75	0.82	6.92	5.57	4.15
MET	0.75	0.72	0.77	6.83	5.81	4.89
TSF	0.70	0.72	0.86	6.70	5.91	3.28

[a]Significant effects in repeated measures analysis of covariance. Treatment Compliance Group: $F = 28.51$, df = 2, 1541, $p < 0.001$; time: $F = 2.75$; df = 3, 4626; $p < 0.05$; Treatment Compliance Group by Treatment Assignment: $F = 3.76$; df = 4, 1541; $p < 0.01$.
[b]Significant effects in ANACOVA. Treatment Compliance Group: $F = 32.74$; df = 2, 1541, $p < 0.001$; Treatment Compliance Group by Treatment Assignment: $F = 3.02$; df = 4, 1541; $p < 0.05$.
Note. Values of the dependent variables are in their original rather than transformed metrics.

factors related to treatment compliance (e.g., motivation) were responsible for the observed declines in alcohol use.

The analyses of compliance and data quality indicators reviewed in this section lead to several conclusions regarding the internal and external validity of the findings. First, the data collected in the trial were very complete. A high proportion of participants complied with the demands of the research protocol throughout the course of the trial, and the level of research participation did not vary as a function of treatment condition. Second, the self-report methods that served as the basis for constructing the primary treatment outcome variables used in the trial appear to have provided sensitive and relatively unbiased measures of drinking behavior. Further, relatively few individual difference factors were related to research compliance or to discrepancies among different sources of drinking data. Third, although the research procedures themselves may have contributed to changes in drinking, it appears unlikely that reductions in alcohol consumption observed in the trial are solely attributable to the effects of taking part in research activities. Collectively, these findings provide support for the internal and external validity of the study results. Finally, the data on research compliance suggest that the methods used to promote completion of study requirements were successful. When compared to other studies of alcoholism treatment, compliance rates in Project MATCH can be considered excellent (Mattson et al., 1998).

Summary and conclusions

This chapter deals with the implementation of the research protocol. A review of the research procedures established for the trial, together with data that permit an evaluation of potential sources of random error and systematic bias, suggests that threats to the internal and external validity of the findings were minimized. Large, diverse participant samples were recruited for the two arms of the trial, and the evidence suggests that these samples did not represent select subsets of the treatment population with a particularly favorable prognosis. Centralized urn randomization procedures, designed to reduce the possibility that random assignment could be compromised, resulted in a relatively equal distribution of key client characteristics across treatment conditions. Reliability of measurement was established within and across CRUs, and the error introduced during data processing and management was found to be virtually nonexistent. Compliance with the research protocol was excellent, and few client factors were found to be related to level of participation. Despite the absence of an untreated control group, no evidence was found to indicate that changes in drinking were solely attributable to artifacts such as attention and assessment experiences. These findings suggest that a high degree of confidence can be placed in the findings presented in subsequent chapters.

6

The matching hypotheses: rationale and predictions

RONALD M. KADDEN, RICHARD LONGABAUGH,
AND PHILIP W. WIRTZ

Twenty-one *a priori* client–treatment matching hypotheses were tested in
Project MATCH, using a design in which participants with a variety of
possible matching attributes were randomly assigned to either
Cognitive–Behavioral Therapy, Motivational Enhancement Therapy, or
Twelve Step Facilitation. Each *a priori* hypothesis was theoretically derived,
and specified the underlying mechanisms through which matching was
presumed to operate. This chapter describes how each hypothesis was
formulated, approved, and tested, as well as its rationale, supporting evidence,
and method for measuring the matching characteristics.

A number of decisions were required at the outset of Project MATCH to
enable assessment of the effectiveness of various matches between clients
and treatments. One of the earliest, and easiest, decisions was that the
matching hypotheses would be specified *a priori*, before providing treatment or collecting data. This was followed by a number of more difficult
decisions. The first was whether clients should be assigned to treatment
prospectively on the basis of the *a priori* hypotheses, or by random assignment. In the absence of independent replication of any prior matching
findings, the Steering Committee opted for a random assignment strategy
that would allow the testing of a number of different *a priori* matching
hypotheses. The Steering Committee also decided that matching should be
tested in relation to different types of *treatment*, rather than to program
types, therapists, or the format, intensity, or duration of treatment.

In order to simplify the research design and interpretability of the
findings, it was decided that all interventions offered in this trial would be
provided on an ambulatory basis. The inpatient sites would offer them as
aftercare following the site's usual treatment regimen, and the outpatient
sites would provide them as the participants' initial exposure to treatment.

These early decisions of the Steering Committee provided the boundary conditions within which the treatments were selected and the matching hypotheses were developed.

Yet another set of decisions related to the form in which the hypotheses would be stated, so that they would all be amenable to common statistical procedures. The ultimate decision was that each hypothesized matching relationship would be tested by comparing regressions of client attributes upon treatment outcomes across different treatments (see Longabaugh et al., 1994b). There would be a separate regression line for each of the treatments being contrasted in a matching hypothesis, and comparisons would be specified in terms of differences between the *slopes* of these regression lines (i.e., as differences in the rates of change of an outcome variable along a client attribute dimension, compared across different treatments). Stated in this way, the hypotheses did not include explicit tests of whether the interactions between the client attribute and the treatments were ordinal (i.e., the regression lines did not cross within the range of values observed for the client matching attribute) or disordinal (i.e., the lines did cross such that one treatment was superior at one end of the attribute and worse at the other end). Nor did the matching hypotheses include mention of the relative positions of the regression lines (i.e., no predictions of treatment main effects were made); the hypotheses only specified comparisons between slopes.

Development of the matching hypotheses

After the treatments were selected, the Steering Committee suggested topical areas that could be considered for possible matching hypotheses. Members with similar interests were invited to form teams to develop specific hypotheses. The first task of the hypothesis teams was to conduct a literature review to identify theoretical and empirical support for a possible match between a client characteristic and the selected treatments. These reviews were summarized in written 'position papers,' which were later expanded to provide the full statement of the proposed hypothesis. A fully developed hypothesis statement included a rationale, description of supportive studies in the literature, a verbal statement of the hypothesis, a mathematical formulation, procedures for operationalizing the matching variable, specification of the dependent variables that would test for matching, and a data analysis plan.

Once an hypothesis was adopted by the Steering Committee, the teams were charged with identifying intervening variables that might explain the mechanisms of action by which the client attribute interacted with the treatment to which it was matched. The resulting 'causal chains' were designed to empirically test the theoretical underpinnings of each matching hypothesis, and to provide information that might help explain the reasons for failure, in case hypotheses were not supported. The statement of the causal chain for a specific matching hypothesis and the plan for testing it required Steering Committee approval, and then became part of the hypothesis document. All of the documents for the various hypotheses were finalized prior to conducting the first analyses of any outcome data.

Approval process

Four criteria were used to choose the hypotheses:

1. An hypothesis had to be based on a clearly conceptualized client attribute that could be readily measured.
2. There had to be prior evidence of matching effects using this client attribute, or evidence of a main effect of the attribute and a theoretical basis for believing that differential matching to one or more of the Project MATCH treatments would be likely.
3. The proposed interaction between the attribute and the treatments had to be likely to have a significant impact on outcome.
4. The client attribute had to be relatively independent of, but not contradictory to, any of the other attributes being considered as matching variables.

As the review process proceeded, a few hypotheses failed to receive Steering Committee approval. Nevertheless, the number of remaining hypotheses was still quite large. As a result, the Steering Committee designated two tiers of *a priori* hypotheses: those that had strong empirical or theoretical support were considered *primary* hypotheses, and those with less support or a weaker rationale were designated *secondary* hypotheses. The primary hypotheses were the main hypotheses of the trial and were analyzed first, whereas the secondaries had a less prominent status and were analyzed later. In a few cases there were alternative ways of conceptualizing or operationalizing a client attribute; in those instances, one version was designated as the primary hypothesis and the other as secondary.

In formulating the hypotheses, the hypothesis teams had to consider which treatments to include in specifying the matching relationship. With three treatments provided in the trial, an hypothesis could specify a matching relationship between a client attribute and one, two, or three of the treatments. It was also possible to specify a match to a combination of two of the treatments in relation to the third one. Each of these possible comparisons was referred to as a contrast. In some instances, the hypothesis team decided to specify only the contrast that they believed had the greatest likelihood of differentially affecting outcome, resulting in hypotheses that included only two of the three treatments.

The final product of this lengthy process was a group of 10 primary and 11 secondary *a priori* matching hypotheses that received Steering Committee approval. Some of them involved multiple contrasts among the three treatments, resulting in over 30 hypothesized contrasts, a number which substantially inflates the risk of a Type I error (i.e., finding a matching effect that resulted from chance variation). One means of correcting for this would be a Bonferroni adjustment, which tests each of the hypotheses at an alpha level (e.g., $p < 0.05$), divided by the total number of hypotheses (Wirtz et al., 1994). However, there was concern that strict application of this method across all of the hypotheses, specified contrasts, and two outcome variables per contrast, would result in an excessively conservative cut-off level for statistical significance that would unduly enhance the likelihood of a Type II error (i.e., accepting the null hypothesis of no differences when in fact a true matching effect had occurred). Because the matching hypotheses were conceived as conceptually independent of one another, it was decided to apply a Bonferroni correction to tests of significance within each hypothesis 'family.' Thus, each of the primary and secondary matching hypotheses was allotted a family-wise Type I error rate of 5%. That value was then halved to take into account the two primary outcome variables (Percent Days Abstinent and Drinks per Drinking Day), and was further reduced if there was more than one proposed contrast for an hypothesis.

The matching hypotheses

Tables 6.1 and 6.2 summarize the primary and secondary *a priori* matching hypotheses, respectively, listing the contrasts that were specified and the means by which the client matching attributes were measured. The rationale and causal chain for each primary and secondary hypothesis are summarized below, with full details provided in a separate monograph devoted to the causal mechanisms behind treatment matching (Longabaugh & Wirtz, 2001).

The primary hypotheses

Alcohol Involvement

The concept of alcohol involvement, reflecting the extent to which one's lifestyle has been influenced by drinking, is more inclusive than the diagnostic criteria for alcohol dependence. It includes elements such as drinking in a sustained fashion, obsession with drinking, and social consequences that may result from drinking. Greater alcohol involvement has been shown to increase the risk of relapse following treatment, and is associated with greater frequency and intensity of drinking (Rounsaville et al., 1987; Horn et al., 1990).

Research at the time the matching hypotheses were conceived suggested that greater treatment intensity is more effective for clients with greater problem severity (Orford et al., 1976). In formulating the alcohol involvement hypothesis, it was assumed that treatments with more therapeutic contact would monitor clients more effectively, detect and respond to relapses more promptly, provide more support for behavior change, be more effective in dealing with low self-efficacy, and create a stronger therapeutic relationship. Therefore, it was predicted that clients with greater alcohol involvement would have better outcomes with the more intensive treatments – Cognitive–Behavioral Therapy (CBT) and Twelve Step Facilitation (TSF) – than with the less intensive Motivational Enhancement Therapy (MET). Alcohol Involvement was assessed by means of the Alcohol Involvement scale of the Alcohol Use Inventory (Horn et al., 1990).

Cognitive Impairment

Alcoholics often have significant impairment of cognitive functioning, even following detoxification (Parsons, 1986), and those with greater impairment show less clinical improvement as a result of treatment (e.g., Donovan et al., 1985). Basic processes such as attention, abstract reasoning, and cognitive flexibility may be impaired in alcoholics (McCrady & Smith, 1986). As a result, they may have difficulty absorbing, processing, generalizing, and applying information that is provided during treatment.

Table 6.1. *Measurement instruments and hypothesized contrasts of slopes or differences between means for each primary matching variable*

Matching variable	Measurement procedure	Hypothesized contrast[a]
Alcohol Involvement[b]	Alcohol Use Inventory	[CBT, TSF] slope > MET slope
Cognitive Impairment[c]	Shipley Institute of Living Scale; Trails B; Symbol–Digit Modalities Test	TSF slope > CBT slope CBT slope > MET slope TSF slope > MET slope
Conceptual Level	Paragraph Completion Method	MET slope > TSF slope
Gender	Self-report question	Female (CBT mean − TSF mean) > male (CBT mean − TSF mean)
Meaning Seeking[b]	Purpose in Life Scale; Seeking of Noetic Goals Scale	TSF slope > [MET, CBT] slope
Motivation	University of Rhode Island Change Assessment Scale	CBT slope > MET slope
Psychiatric Severity[c]	Addiction Severity Index: Psychiatric Severity Scale	CBT slope > MET slope CBT slope > TSF slope
Sociopathy[c]	California Psychological Inventory – Socialization Scale	CBT slope > MET slope CBT slope > TSF slope TSF slope > MET slope
Support for Drinking[c]	Important People and Activities Interview	CBT slope > MET slope TSF slope > MET slope
Typology[b]	Combination of measures (see text)	Type B ([CBT, TSF] mean − MET mean) > Type A ([CBT, TSF] mean − MET mean)

[a]The hypothesized contrasts predict differences in slopes of the regression lines for each treatment on outcome as a function of client attribute. With the exception of the Gender and Typology attributes (which take on only discrete values), all contrasts take the form: the difference between the first treatment and the second becomes more positive (or less negative) with increasing values of the attribute. The Gender and Typology attributes take the form: the difference in means between the treatments is greater at one level of the attribute than at the other. Hypotheses did not test whether interactions were ordinal or disordinal.

[b]The rationale underlying the Alcohol Involvement, Meaning Seeking, and Typology hypotheses assumes that, because of similar active ingredients involved in the hypothesized matching effect, the two treatments are not different in their effects. Therefore, they were combined into a single condition that was then contrasted with the third treatment.

[c]Cognitive Impairment and Sociopathy each involved three hypothesized treatment contrasts. Therefore, the Bonferroni family-wide correction was applied to divide the alpha level by 3 for each of these attributes. Support for Drinking and Psychiatric Severity each involved two hypothesized contrasts; thus each of these contrasts involved dividing the alpha level by 2. All other attributes involved single contrasts.

Table 6.2. *Measurement instruments and hypothesized contrasts of slopes or differences between means for secondary matching hypotheses*

Matching variable	Measurement procedure	Hypothesized contrast[a]
Alcohol Dependence[c]	Ethanol Dependence Syndrome Scale	TSF slope > CBT slope
		TSF slope > MET slope
Anger[b]	Trait Anger Scale	MET slope > [CBT, TSF] slope
Antisocial Personality Disorder[c]	Computerized Diagnostic Interview Schedule	CBT slope > MET slope
		TSF slope > MET slope
		CBT slope > TSF slope
Interpersonal Dependency[b]	Interpersonal Dependency Inventory, Assertion of Autonomy Subscale	[CBT, MET] slope > TSF slope
Psychopathology DSM-III-R Axis I Diagnosis[c]	Computerized Diagnostic Interview Schedule	CBT slope > MET slope
		CBT slope > TSF slope
Prior Engagement in Alcoholics Anonymous[b]	AA Involvement Scale	TSF slope > [CBT, MET] slope
Readiness to Change[b]	Stages of Change Readiness and Treatment Eagerness Scale	[CBT, TSF] slope > MET slope
Religiosity[b]	Religious Background and Behavior Questionnaire	TSF slope > [CBT, MET] slope
Self-efficacy[c] Confidence	Alcohol Abstinence Self-efficacy Scale: Confidence in Abstinence subscale	MET slope > CBT slope
		MET slope > TSF slope
Temptation minus Confidence	Difference between Temptation and Confidence subscale scores	TSF slope > MET slope
Social Functioning[c]	Psychosocial Functioning Inventory; Drinker Inventory of Consequences	TSF slope > CBT slope
		MET slope > CBT slope

[a] The hypothesized contrasts predict differences in slopes of the regression lines for each treatment on outcome as a function of client attribute. All contrasts take the form: the difference between the first treatment and the second becomes more positive (or less negative) with increasing values on the attribute. Hypotheses did not test whether interactions were ordinal or disordinal.
[b] The rationale underlying the Anger, Religiosity, Interpersonal Dependency, Prior Engagement in AA, and Readiness to Change hypotheses assumes that, because of similar active ingredients involved in the hypothesized matching effect, the two treatments are not different in their effects. Therefore, they were combined into a single condition that was then contrasted with the third treatment.
[c] The Alcohol Dependence, Antisocial Personality Disorder, Psychopathology, Self-efficacy and Social Functioning hypotheses each involved two or three treatment contrasts. Therefore, the Bonferroni family-wide correction was applied to divide the alpha level by the number of contrasts for each of these attributes. All other attributes involved single contrasts.

It was therefore anticipated that those with greater cognitive impairment would have poorer outcomes, regardless of treatment type. With respect to client–treatment matching, it was hypothesized that greater treatment structure, intensity, and duration would benefit those who were more cognitively impaired. Such clients would benefit more from either CBT or TSF, than from MET, whereas less impaired clients would do equally well in all of the treatments. Based on findings that cognitively impaired alcoholics had comparatively poorer outcomes in cognitive–behavioral treatments (Kadden et al., 1989; Jaffe et al., 1996), it was also predicted that TSF, with its emphasis on repeated, straightforward messages (slogans), and the social support of AA meetings, would produce superior outcomes in comparison to CBT.

Cognitive Impairment was operationalized as a combination of three different measures. Scores from the Shipley Institute of Living Abstraction subscale (Shipley, 1940), the Trail Making Test Part B (Reitan, 1958) and the Symbol Digit Modalities Test (Smith, 1973) were entered into a principal components analysis with varimax rotation, which yielded a single factor. On the basis of this analysis, a composite Cognitive Impairment Index was developed, which was the sum of unit-weighted standardized scores for the Shipley Abstraction T-score, Trails B total time, and the number of correct responses (in 90 s) on the Symbol Digit Test.

Conceptual Level

Conceptual Level refers to a person's cognitive style of relating to the environment. People with a low conceptual level tend to function most effectively in structured environments. Those high on this dimension do best with little structure and maximal independence. In tests of matching based on this dimension, McLachlan (1972, 1974) found that alcoholic clients who were matched either to therapists with a similar conceptual level or to the degree of structure of the aftercare they received had outcomes that were superior to clients who were mismatched to their therapist or to the structure of their aftercare. The McLachlan (1972) paper was one of the first in the literature reporting successful matching for alcoholics. The hypothesis, as formulated in Project MATCH, was that those clients with a lower conceptual level would have better outcomes if treated with TSF than with MET, because TSF is a more structured treatment, and it teaches clients to rely on external structures – Alcoholics Anonymous (AA) meetings and a sponsor. On the other hand, it was predicted that those with higher conceptual level would have superior outcomes with MET, which urges clients to make decisions for themselves. Conceptual Level was operationalized by means of the Paragraph Completion Method (Hunt et al., 1978).

Gender

Women tend to attribute their drinking to external stressors and negative moods more often than men (Babor et al., 1991), are more likely to seek treatment for physical, emotional, and marital/family problems (Duckert, 1987), and are more often characterized as passive, dependent, and lacking self-esteem (Beckman, 1978). Consequently, it has been suggested that treatments focused on coping skills and relapse prevention should be particularly effective for women (Institute of Medicine, 1990), and a meta-analytic study found that female alcoholics tended to fare better in behaviorally oriented therapies, compared to males who benefited more from inpatient treatment that included psychotherapy, milieu therapy, and AA (Jarvis, 1992). Within Project MATCH, CBT dealt most directly with factors that tend to characterize alcoholic women and may contribute to their drinking. TSF, on the other hand, does not address these factors explicitly, and the confrontational style of AA may be contraindicated for females who traditionally assume non-confrontational, conciliatory roles. Thus, it was hypothesized that females treated in CBT would have better outcomes than those treated in TSF. The prediction regarding males was that the difference in outcomes between CBT and TSF would be less than for females.

Meaning Seeking

A common recommendation to clients with drinking problems is that they get involved in AA. A meta-analytic review (Emrick et al., 1993) suggests that participation in AA is, in fact, associated with favorable treatment outcome, although no single predictor of AA affiliation explained as much as 10% of the variance in AA attendance. According to the AA 'Big Book,' those who are most likely to benefit from AA are those who have 'hit bottom,' a concept involving both demoralization and a willingness to accept help. Demoralization includes the feeling that life has lost meaning, often accompanied by a desire to find more meaning in life. In the present study, a combination of two instruments was used to assess these two aspects of demoralization. One was Crumbaugh and Maholick's (1976) Purpose in Life (PIL) scale, designed to assess current sense of meaning in life. This was used to provide an operational measure of 'hitting bottom.' The other instrument was the Seeking of Noetic Goals (SONG) scale (Crumbaugh, 1977b), designed to assess desire for, and efforts to seek, greater meaning in life. This scale was used to assess the AA concept of willingness to change. To capture both elements in a single score, the PIL score was subtracted from the SONG score, producing a continuum ranging from a low sense of meaning combined with a strong desire to find meaning, at one extreme, to a strong current sense of meaning combined with a low desire to find greater meaning, at the other. It was predicted that those with high scores on this derived measure (low meaning and strong desire to find meaning) would have better outcomes if treated in TSF, because its primary goal was to foster AA involvement, and poorer outcomes with the other two interventions.

Motivation

Motivation to change drinking behavior was conceptualized in terms of the stages of change construct, which identifies five steps, or stages, that individuals typically pass through in the course of changing their behavior (Prochaska & DiClemente, 1984). People in the early stages have difficulty engaging in treatment and changing their behavior, whereas those in the later stages are already engaged in the process of change (Prochaska et al., 1992). It was hypothesized that the motivational strategies that are the hallmark of MET would be particularly effective with clients in the early stages of change. It was expected that CBT would be less effective with these clients because of its action-oriented approach, which might be premature for poorly motivated clients. No predictions were made regarding treatment differences for highly motivated participants; it was thought that they might do equally well in all treatments.

Stage of change was assessed by the Alcohol Stages of Change version of the University of Rhode Island Change Assessment (URICA), which measures attitudes typically associated with the different stages of change (DiClemente & Hughes, 1990). The subscales of this instrument combine to form a second-order factor, Readiness to Change, which was used as the indicator of motivation in this hypothesis.

Psychiatric Severity

The high prevalence of comorbid psychiatric problems among clients with substance-use disorders (Regier et al., 1990) adversely affects treatment outcomes (McLellan et al., 1984; Rounsaville et al., 1987). In addition, interactions have been found between the degree of psychiatric severity and types of treatment (Woody et al., 1984; Kadden et al., 1989).

Strategies to treat psychopathology were incorporated into CBT as elective sessions to help clients cope with social anxiety, depression, and anger. In contrast, TSF and MET provided no specific interventions for clients with psychopathology. MET's brevity precluded a focus on problems beyond drinking and it was thought to be too demanding for those with significant psychopathology, whereas TSF made the assumption that mild psychopathology would improve with abstinence and that severe psychopathology would require referral to a mental health professional. An additional consideration is that more intensive treatment is often recommended for alcoholics with a high degree of psychopathology. The Psychiatric Severity hypothesis was based on the differences among treatments in both content and intensity, predicting superior outcomes for the more psychiatrically impaired clients treated in CBT as compared to MET. A second *a priori* contrast tested treatments equated on intensity, to allow an interpretation of matching effects related to the content of treatment. The prediction was that CBT would be superior to TSF for clients who manifested greater psychopathology.

This matching variable was assessed by means of the Psychiatric Severity composite score of the Addiction Severity Index (ASI; McLellan et al., 1980), which measures psychiatric symptomatology across a number of problem areas, especially depression and anxiety.

Sociopathy

The term sociopathy refers to aspects of personality such as lack of remorse, incapacity for love, superficial charm, egocentricity, and poverty in affective reactions. The term has also come to include behavior patterns such as aggressiveness, repeated lying, recklessness, and failure to honor obligations. Researchers have found associations among sociopathy, alcoholism (Lewis et al., 1983), and poor treatment outcomes (Rounsaville et al., 1987). A matching study found superior outcomes for sociopathic alcoholics who had been treated with CBT, as compared to an interactional approach (Kadden et al., 1989; Cooney et al., 1991). In light of this evidence, sociopathy was selected as a promising matching variable.

Sociopaths often lack appropriate social skills, may be unable to develop good therapeutic relationships (e.g., Gerstley et al., 1989), and are often angry. It was expected that sociopaths would benefit from treatment structure (Frosch, 1983) and from anger management training, but would not be likely to get involved in AA because of their difficulties in forming interpersonal relationships. Based on these considerations, it was predicted that sociopathic clients would have better outcomes with CBT as opposed to MET, because CBT does not require a working alliance with the therapist, is a more structured therapy, and teaches skills to manage anger. It was further hypothesized that TSF would be more effective for sociopathic clients than MET because of its greater structure. Finally, CBT was hypothesized to be superior to TSF for sociopathic clients because it would teach skills to manage anger and because it does not require AA attendance, which would be difficult for sociopathic clients to sustain. Sociopathy was assessed by means of the Socialization scale of the California Psychological Inventory (Gough, 1987; see also Cooney et al., 1990).

Social Support for Drinking

A social network oriented towards activities that involve the use of alcohol is likely to have a deleterious effect on treatment outcome (Longabaugh & Beattie, 1985; Longabaugh et al., 1993). An obvious question for matching research is whether interventions targeted towards destructive social networks will have a positive impact on drinking outcomes. Two of the treatments in Project MATCH were considered likely to influence social support for drinking: TSF promotes involvement in AA, which provides a ready-made social system strongly supportive of abstinence, and CBT teaches drink refusal and other interpersonal skills that could be used to cope with an alcohol-oriented social network. MET, on the other hand, has no specific features that directly address vulnerability to a pre-existing network supportive of drinking. The Support for Drinking hypothesis therefore predicted that clients whose social network was more supportive of drinking would fare worse in MET than in either TSF or CBT. No prediction was made for clients whose social network was not supportive of drinking. Network support for drinking was assessed by means of the

Important People and Activities interview, which identifies the important people in a client's social network, their drinking habits, and their behavior towards the client's drinking or abstinence (Clifford & Longabaugh, 1991).

Typology

Alcoholism appears to be a multiply determined problem, with biological, psychological, and social factors all contributing to its etiology (Tarter, 1983). This view has stimulated efforts to classify alcoholics into subtypes having similar etiological profiles. Identification of subtypes raises the question of whether they would benefit from treatments designed to accommodate their particular needs. Babor et al. (1992) utilized cluster analysis to identify two subtypes, one of which had better outcomes with interactional group therapy, whereas the other fared better with cognitive–behavioral group therapy (Litt et al., 1992). The former cluster, 'Type A,' is characterized by later onset of drinking, fewer indicators of vulnerability, less psychiatric disturbance, more benign alcohol-related problems, and better prognosis. The latter cluster, 'Type B,' is characterized by a family history of alcoholism, childhood conduct problems, early onset of drinking, rapid progression of drinking-related problems, more psychiatric disturbance, greater alcoholism symptom severity, and poor prognosis. Project MATCH provided an opportunity to further explore the matching potential of this typology with different treatments. It was hypothesized that Type B clients would have poorer outcomes overall, but would fare better in the CBT and TSF interventions because of their greater structure and intensity (12 sessions), and because of the skills training aspect of CBT. It was also predicted that Type A clients would have better outcomes with MET, preferring the autonomy that this approach allows and making good use of the therapeutic relationship that was expected to develop in MET. Based on previous research (Babor et al., 1992), the typology was operationalized by means of five measures:

1. percent of first-degree relatives positive for alcohol dependence (McLellan et al., 1992);
2. the MacAndrew (1965) Alcoholism scale from the Minnesota Multiphasic Personality Inventory (MMPI);
3. the total score from the Ethanol Dependence Syndrome scale (Babor, 1996);

4. physical effects of drinking from the Drinker Inventory of Consequences (Miller et al., 1995b);
5. the antisocial personality disorder symptom count from the Computerized Diagnostic Interview Schedule (Blouin et al., 1988).

Participants who scored above established medians in at least three of the five domains were classified as Type B alcoholics (high vulnerability, high severity), and all others were classified as Type A.

The secondary hypotheses

Alcohol Dependence

The alcohol dependence syndrome (Edwards & Gross, 1976) is a set of interrelated symptoms that include neuroadaptation to alcohol, cognitive supports for heavy drinking, and impaired control over alcohol intake (Edwards, 1986; Babor et al., 1987b). The syndrome has been validated across cultures (Hall et al., 1993) and predicts the rapidity of reinstatement of dependence symptoms following a relapse (Babor et al., 1987a). Orford et al. (1976) found evidence for matching clients to different treatment intensities based on their level of dependence, although a re-analysis of their data has called that conclusion into question (Edwards & Taylor, 1994).

Despite its similarity to the alcohol involvement variable, the two matching hypotheses made somewhat different predictions. The Alcohol Involvement (primary) hypothesis was based on the expectation that more intensive treatment would be needed to produce good outcomes for clients with greater alcohol involvement. The Alcohol Dependence (secondary) hypothesis, on the other hand, made matching predictions based on differences in the content of the three Project MATCH therapies. Severely dependent clients were expected to have better outcomes with TSF (because of its emphasis on total abstinence and loss of control), worse outcomes with CBT (because coping skills training may not provide adequate preparation to deal with the rapid reinstatement of dependence after a relapse), and worse outcomes with MET (because clients may be tempted to pursue a moderate drinking goal or may require more than just client-generated recovery strategies). In contrast, clients with mild dependence were expected to: (1) have better outcomes with CBT because they could more effectively utilize newly acquired skills to cope with a lapse; (2) have equally good outcomes with MET because they would have a reasonable chance of success if they pursued a moderate drinking goal; and (3) do poorly with TSF because its emphasis on loss of control after any alcohol consumption would not be consistent with their personal experience. Accordingly, this hypothesis was tested with two *a priori* contrasts, one comparing TSF and CBT, and the other comparing TSF and MET. Dependence severity was assessed using the Ethanol Dependence Scale (Hesselbrock et al., 1983; Babor, 1996).

Anger

Anger is a common problem among alcoholics seeking treatment (Deffenbacher et al., 1994). Clients often deny that their anger is a problem, and are prone to defensive reactions that render them resistant to treatment and interfere with forming a working alliance with the therapist. Therapist behaviors such as confrontation, directiveness, and teaching are additional factors that can increase client resistance (Patterson & Forgatch, 1985). Among the Project MATCH treatments, MET used specific strategies to defuse resistance and avoid confrontation. MET therapists were trained to express empathy, support self-efficacy, enhance motivation, and encourage clients to make choices in therapy. It was therefore hypothesized that clients high in anger would have better outcomes after treatment in MET than in either CBT or TSF, which are more didactic and directive. No differences among treatments were predicted for clients low in anger. Anger was measured by means of the State–Trait Anger Expression Inventory (Spielberger, 1988), which assesses anger as both a situational response (state) and as a disposition (trait). Only the trait aspect of anger was used to test the hypothesis.

Antisocial Personality Disorder

Antisocial Personality Disorder (ASPD) is a clinical diagnosis assigned to individuals who meet behaviorally based criteria that encompass a pattern of irresponsible and antisocial behavior beginning in early adolescence and continuing into adulthood. This secondary hypothesis sought to determine whether a diagnosis of ASPD would provide a better clinical basis for matching than the continuous measure of sociopathy (CPI-So) that was employed to test a primary hypothesis. Successful matching to the ASPD categorical diagnosis would be advantageous because it is part of the American Psychiatric Association's (1987) *Diagnostic and Statistical*

Manual (DSM), which is well understood by clinicians. Longabaugh et al. (1994a) found that clients with an ASPD diagnosis had better outcomes if matched to cognitive–behavioral therapy.

In every respect, this hypothesis was identical to the Sociopathy primary hypothesis. It involved the same three contrasts and made the same predictions. The anticipated contrasts for clients with ASPD, as for sociopathic clients, were that CBT and TSF would be more effective than MET, and that CBT would be superior to TSF. The only difference is that the client attribute was operationalized by means of the DSM-III-R diagnosis of ASPD as determined by the Computerized Diagnostic Interview Schedule (C-DIS) (Blouin et al., 1988; Robins et al., 1989), rather than by the continuous CPI-So measure.

Interpersonal Dependency

Studies have shown a positive association between alcoholism and interpersonal dependency (Bornstein, 1992). Although dependency-related behaviors seem to increase with the development of alcohol problems and therefore may not be an important etiologic factor, the presence of interpersonal dependency at the time of treatment may nevertheless affect outcome and may interact with type of treatment. The AA approach attempts to deal with the dependency needs of alcoholics, seeking to redirect them towards the AA group and towards a 'higher power.' Some studies have shown a relationship between dependency needs and affiliation with AA (Ogborne & Glaser, 1981). The CBT and MET approaches to treatment, on the other hand, ask the individual to assume responsibility for self-management and decision making. It was therefore hypothesized that clients with high interpersonal dependency would benefit most from the TSF intervention, as compared with CBT and MET. On the other hand, clients with low interpersonal dependency are likely to be self-reliant and have less need for the support and nurturance provided by self-help groups. It was predicted that they would fare less well in TSF, and better in CBT or MET, which emphasize self-management. Interpersonal Dependency was measured using the Assertion of Autonomy subscale of the Interpersonal Dependency Inventory (Hirschfeld et al., 1977). This particular subscale ranges from dependence on others' approval for self-esteem, at the low end, to indifference to others' evaluation, at the high end.

Psychopathology

This hypothesis is an alternative version of the Psychiatric Severity primary hypothesis, in this case employing DSM-III-R Axis I diagnosis as the matching variable. Because diagnostic categories such as depression and anxiety are more familiar to clinicians than the ASI measure of Psychiatric Severity, it was felt that matching based on this variable might be more clinically useful. However, it was assigned secondary hypothesis status because prior research had found matching to the ASI measure of Psychiatric Severity but not to clinical diagnoses, and because of the greater statistical power inherent in the ASI continuous variable as opposed to discrete diagnostic categories. The predictions for this hypothesis, and the reasoning behind them, were similar to the Psychiatric Severity hypothesis: clients with a comorbid anxiety or affective disorder would have better outcomes if treated in CBT rather than in either TSF or MET.

The matching variable for this hypothesis was operationalized according to the lifetime diagnostic criteria for any anxiety or affective disorder, as assessed by the C-DIS, with the additional requirement that one or more relevant symptoms must have occurred in the past 6 months.

Prior Engagement in Alcoholics Anonymous

Many people who seek alcoholism treatment have had prior exposure to AA. In the context of the present study, it was predicted that those who had more involvement in AA would have a greater commitment to and more faith in that approach. As a result, they would fare better in the AA-oriented TSF treatment than in either of the others, which took a neutral stance with regard to AA participation. It was therefore hypothesized that, with increasing levels of prior AA involvement, clients would have better outcomes if treated in TSF than in CBT or MET. Prior engagement in AA was operationalized by means of the Alcoholics Anonymous Involvement scale (Tonigan et al., 1996a).

Readiness to Change

This is an alternative version of the Motivation primary hypothesis. In that hypothesis, motivation was assessed by means of the URICA scale, which was developed to assess stages of change across a broad array of problems, employing items framed in general terms. An alternative scale, the Stages of Change Readiness and Treatment Eagerness Scale (SOCRATES), was designed to provide a drinking-specific.assessment of the same stages of change as assessed by the URICA (Miller & Tonigan, 1996). However, unlike the URICA, factor analyses of the SOCRATES consistently yield only three factors, which have been labeled Ambivalence, Recognition, and Taking steps. The Recognition factor was chosen as the indicator of Readiness to Change, for this secondary hypothesis, based on its item loadings. In framing the Readiness to Change secondary hypothesis, it was predicted that less motivated clients treated in MET would have better outcomes than similar clients treated in CBT or TSF.

Religiosity

The Meaning Seeking primary hypothesis attempted to account for an important aspect of the crisis that occurs when an alcoholic 'hits bottom,' thus making AA the logical choice for help. However, that hypothesis did not seek to account for religiosity, an additional factor that might predict success in the spiritually oriented AA program, which involves faith in God or a 'higher power,' surrender to God's will, and prayer or meditation. A previous study reported a modest relationship between the extent of one's religious and spiritual activities and AA affiliation (Fichter, 1982). It was therefore hypothesized that those with greater religiosity would benefit more from the TSF intervention, which emphasized AA participation, than from the other two treatment approaches. Those with little religiosity were not expected to derive as much benefit from exposure to TSF. The Religious Background and Behavior (RBB) questionnaire was developed for this study to assess the extent of religious beliefs, experiences, and practices (Connors et al., 1996).

Self-efficacy

Self-efficacy is a personal evaluation of one's ability to perform a particular behavior. It is central to Marlatt's conceptualization of the relapse process (Marlatt & Gordon, 1985), and has been assessed in terms of efficacy for coping (Annis & Davis, 1989) and efficacy to abstain from drinking (DiClemente et al., 1994a). In Project MATCH it was hypothesized that clients with high self-efficacy, or 'confidence,' would do better in MET because it encouraged them to draw upon their own resources and formulate their own change plan. On the other hand, clients low in self-efficacy were expected to fare better in either CBT or TSF because of their focus, respectively, on skills development or external support, neither of which requires pre-existing self-efficacy.

An alternative hypothesis relating to self-efficacy proposed that clients with low self-efficacy who report high levels of temptation to drink would be particularly vulnerable to relapse. These individuals may feel overwhelmed by the personal responsibility required to profit from MET, and would fare better with the support and reliance on a higher power offered by TSF.

The first formulation of the Self-efficacy hypothesis was operationalized by means of the Confidence subscale of the Alcohol Abstinence Self-Efficacy (AASE) scale (DiClemente et al., 1994a). To test the second formulation, a score was derived for each subject consisting of his/her AASE temptation subscale score minus the confidence score. Clients with a large positive difference (high temptation combined with low confidence) were expected to have better outcomes with TSF.

Social Functioning

Clients with relatively high levels of social functioning prior to alcoholism treatment are likely to have good treatment outcomes (e.g., Edwards et al., 1988; Emrick et al., 1993). One way to improve treatment outcomes would be to reduce the disadvantage of poor social functioning. One study showed that cognitive–behavioral treatment can be particularly helpful to clients with deficits in relapse-related social skills (Kadden et al., 1992b), although another study failed to demonstrate such an effect (Rohsenow et al., 1991). In Project MATCH, the CBT intervention contained both core and elective sessions that targeted alcohol-related as well as general social skills deficits, whereas TSF and MET both required some degree of social functioning for their success, and neither provided specific remediation in this regard. Therefore, it was hypothesized that clients with less adequate social functioning would benefit more from CBT than from the other two treatments, and that the greater the client's level of social functioning, the more he or she would benefit from TSF or MET.

To construct the Social Functioning variable, clients' scores on the Social Behavior subscale of the Psychosocial Functioning Inventory (Feragne et al., 1983) and the Social Relationship subscale of the Drinker Inventory of Consequences (Miller et al., 1995b) were each converted to scores with a range between 0 and 1. These two converted scores were then summed to yield a Social Functioning Index ranging from 0 to 2. High scores on this derived index identified persons who functioned well in terms of their social behavior and who had no negative social consequences due to alcohol use, whereas those with low scores had poor social behavior and considerable negative social consequences due to alcohol.

Summary

Given the number of previously reported matching studies based on small samples and different research approaches, there was a need to evaluate competing matching hypotheses across different treatment settings in a large multisite study sample. Project MATCH specified a set of *a priori* matching hypotheses that were tested by randomly assigning clients to one of three different treatments. This strategy allowed the evaluation of a large number of matching hypotheses within the same data set, as well as the identification of the success profiles of different treatment groups. By assuring pre-treatment equivalence of groups, differences in response could be attributed to treatment effects (Miller & Cooney, 1994).

It was considered important to specify the theory underlying each of the matching hypotheses. This assured that adequate measures would be used to test each hypothesis and the mediating factors that were presumed to account for matching effects. In addition, specifying and assessing the theoretical assumptions provided a framework for interpreting the findings (Longabaugh et al., 1994b). By paying close attention to these issues, the Project MATCH Steering Committee assured a rigorous test of 21 matching hypotheses that were specified *a priori*, as well as an opportunity to explore other matching effects not predicted in advance.

Part II
Findings

7

Primary treatment outcomes and matching effects: Outpatient arm

ROBERT STOUT, FRANCES K. DEL BOCA, JOSEPH CARBONARI,
ROBERT RYCHTARIK, MARK D. LITT, AND NED L. COONEY

As described in Chapter 2, Project MATCH tested matching hypotheses across three treatments in two parallel studies: one with clients recruited directly into outpatient clinics, the other with clients receiving aftercare following the completion of inpatient or day-hospital treatment. This chapter summarizes the major findings for the Outpatient arm. The main effects of the three treatments, as well as matching effects, are presented for the two primary outcome measures, Percent Days Abstinent and Drinks per Drinking Day. The results of analyses testing the causal mechanisms responsible for matching effects are also described. The major findings can be summarized as follows. (1) There were considerable reductions in the frequency and intensity of drinking that followed enrollment in Project MATCH, decreases that were sustained over a 3-year period. (2) There were no consistent and clinically meaningful differences in the efficacy of the three treatments found in the analyses of the primary outcome measures. (3) Only three of the 21 *a priori* matching hypotheses (Psychiatric Severity; Support for Drinking, and Anger) received unqualified support, and the matching effects for these attributes tended to vary as a function of drinking outcome and analysis time frame.

Direct outpatient counseling is one of the most popular models for delivering alcoholism treatment services. In both arms of Project MATCH, participants received the same three treatments (see Chapters 2 and 4). In the Outpatient arm, however, these treatments were delivered as the primary rehabilitation modality, whereas in the Aftercare arm clients received these same therapies only after completing a course of treatment in an inpatient or day-hospital setting. At the time Project MATCH began enrollment, both outpatient approaches (direct admission to outpatient treatment and outpatient treatment as aftercare) were popular in the USA. As the study progressed, however, managed care and cost-containment pressures progressively and dramatically reduced the use of expensive inpatient and day-hospital settings in favor of outpatient services. Although the alcohol treatment delivery system continues to evolve, and inpatient and day-hospital programs have by no means vanished, outpatient care has become much more accepted as a first approach to treating alcohol problems. Thus, the findings from the Outpatient arm, initially reported in four articles (Project MATCH Research Group, 1997a, 1997b, 1998a, 1998b), have special relevance to the emerging alcoholism treatment system. There are also theoretical reasons for interest in treatment matching in outpatient settings. Matching effects might be expected to be strongest where the experimental treatment is the primary intervention. Differential effects from experimental treatments might be diluted in clients who have received large doses of prior treatment.

This chapter describes the statistical analysis approach used in both arms of Project MATCH and summarizes the major results for the Outpatient study. Findings for the Aftercare arm are presented in Chapter 8. The results include treatment and matching attribute main effects, as well as *a priori* treatment matching hypothesis tests for measures of the frequency and intensity of drinking, the two primary treatment outcome measures (see Chapters 3 and 6). In addition, results of analyses designed to test the mechanisms that underlie treatment matching effects (i.e., causal chain analyses) are summarized.

Method

Clinical Research Units and participants

Five of the participating sites (located in Albuquerque, New Mexico; Buffalo, New York; Farmington, Connecticut; Milwaukee, Wisconsin; and West Haven, Connecticut) recruited clients for the Outpatient arm. Participants were recruited directly from the community through advertisements and from outpatient treatment centers. With limited exceptions, the sample was broadly representative of the kinds of clients seen in outpatient treatment programs nationally (see Chapter 5 for a detailed discussion of sample representativeness). On average, clients were 39 years of age; 72% were male, and 80% were Caucasian. A majority (64%) described themselves as single, and almost half (49%) were not employed. Virtually all participants (95%) were alcohol dependent; on average, they drank on more than 4 days a week and, on days when they drank, consumed an average of 13.5 standard drinks (approximately 200 g of ethanol). Many (44%) also used illegal substances, primarily marijuana, in addition to alcohol. Although they were recruited directly into outpatient treatment, almost half (45%) had previously received treatment for alcohol problems (see Chapter 5 for a more detailed description of the Outpatient sample).

Primary outcome measures

Two drinking behavior measures, one of drinking frequency, Percent Days Abstinent (PDA), and the other of intensity, average Drinks per Drinking Day (DDD), were selected *a priori* to serve as primary indicators of treatment outcome (see Babor et al., 1994; and Chapter 3). To study the relatively rapid changes anticipated during treatment (months 1–3), outcome measures were computed for each of the 12 weeks. For the post-treatment analyses, however, outcomes were summarized on a monthly basis. Both the within-treatment and post-treatment analyses therefore involved 12 time points (weeks in one case, months in the other). Alcohol outcomes such as these are prone to substantial departures from normality because of skewness, as well as floor and ceiling effects. Preliminary analyses indicated that an arcsin transformation for PDA, and a square-root transformation for DDD, improved the distribution of these variables.

Statistical analyses

Separate outcome analyses were performed for three time periods: (1) months 1–3 (the 12-week treatment phase); (2) months 4–15 (the 12-month post-treatment follow-up period); and (3) months 37–39 (the 3-year follow-up assessment time window). The reason for separating the first two periods was to have one set of analyses on the effects of treatment as ongoing therapy and another examining outcomes after the experimental treatment ended. Moreover, within-treatment outcome analyses could be directly related to treatment process data. At the 3-year follow-up point, it was possible to assess the persistence of outcomes seen in months 4–15 and to test the durability of any significant main effects, as well as any matching results.

Within-treatment and post-treatment analyses

In the analyses for the first two time frames (i.e., months 1–3 and months 4–15), individual differences in response to treatment were modeled as a

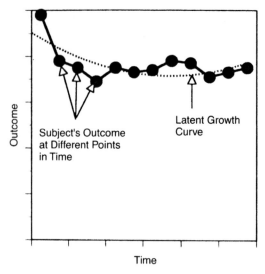

Figure 7.1 A latent growth curve showing a single subject's outcome at different points in time.

multi-level 'latent growth process.' Multi-level latent growth curve analysis is one application of the more general technique of hierarchical linear modeling (HLM; Bryk & Raudenbush, 1987). (A detailed rationale for this approach is given in Carbonari et al., 1994.) Briefly, in a latent growth analysis, temporal variations in outcome (month-to-month or week-to-week) are treated as noise, and the analysis focuses on long-term change. The way this process works is illustrated in Figure 7.1. Data values for individual time points are represented by symbols (blackened circles); the dotted line is the latent growth curve fitted through these data points. Parameter estimates of *individual* change curves (e.g., intercept, linear growth over time, quadratic growth over time) become the dependent variables, and the analysis focuses on how these parameter values are influenced by factors such as client attributes and treatment.

Figure 7.2 shows the three kinds of effects that the latent growth analyses were designed to detect. Treatment or matching variables might affect outcome by shifting the overall level of outcome as shown in the left panel. Alternatively, these effects might grow progressively larger or smaller as indicated in the center panel, or the effects might even change direction over time, as shown on the right. Whereas effects even more complex than these are theoretically possible, they are unlikely to be of

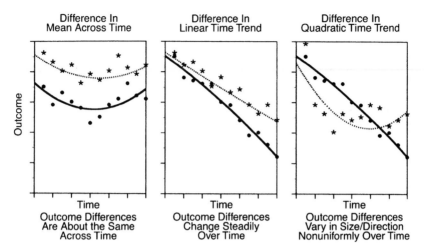

Figure 7.2 Latent growth curves of three different outcome effects across time.

clinical interest. Preliminary model fitting analyses suggested that quadratic curves would be sufficient to account for the effects in the Project MATCH data. The SAS PROC MIXED procedure was used for these analyses (SAS Institute, 1992).

The statistical technique was applied to one outcome variable at a time. Each matching variable was also analyzed independently. There was a Bonferroni adjustment for the number of hypotheses in a 'family' (i.e., pertaining to a specific matching attribute). For example, if there were three hypotheses relating to a single matching variable, each of these hypotheses would be tested at a corrected level of 0.05/3. Because there were two outcome variables, the alpha level was further corrected by a factor of two. The rationale for using a Bonferroni adjustment within, but not across, hypothesis families was that the latter would produce an excessively conservative test and therefore an inflated Type II error rate.

Covariates

There is no consensus about what should be covaried in analyses of treatment outcome. From one perspective, only baseline drinking should be covaried, in which case the approach is similar to analyses of pre–post change in drinking behavior. No other covariates should be needed if randomization has been successful in producing approximately equivalent groups. Another point of view holds that, whereas randomization may produce approximately equivalent groups, it is still prudent to covary measures that may potentially have important effects on outcome. Covarying for these additional factors may reduce noise variance and may improve power. A set of potential nondrinking covariates was selected from the literature for use in the Project MATCH analyses. These were screened in preliminary analyses for distribution properties, missing data, and associations with other potential covariates.

In addition, a special class of covariate, namely site effect terms representing the Clinical Research Units (CRUs), needed to be included to take into account potential intersite variations in client populations and environments that were difficult to measure in advance. Such effects are sometimes seen in multisite trials like Project MATCH, and the latent growth analyses included CRU-related terms. The models controlled for CRU main effects (overall differences in outcome across sites), CRU by treatment interactions (variations across sites in which treatments are more efficacious), CRU by matching variable interactions (variations in the effect of a matching attribute across sites), and CRU by matching variable by treatment interactions (variations in matching effects across sites). These terms not only reduce noise variance (e.g., CRU main effects), but also test the generalizability of matching results across the diverse sites in the sample.

To determine the sensitivity of the major analyses to the selection of covariates, the results were compared using three different levels of covariates: (1) no covariates other than baseline drinking; (2) baseline drinking and CRU terms only (including site main effect and interaction terms); and (3) baseline drinking, CRU terms, and the *a priori* covariate set previously selected. For the most part, there was little difference in the results of the three sets of analyses. Because of the presence of CRU by treatment interactions (see below), it was considered advisable to include site terms in all major analyses. Because there was no appreciable gain in statistical power from using the additional covariates, the baseline drinking and site terms seemed to represent the most parsimonious and effective covariate set. All the latent growth analyses reported in this volume, unless otherwise specified, involve these 'level 2' covariates.

A priori hypothesis tests

The statistical analyses for *a priori* primary and secondary matching hypotheses (detailed in Chapter 6) tested for an interaction effect between the matching variable and different treatment conditions – an attribute by treatment interaction (ATI). There were three indicators of potential matching effects in the latent growth analyses. The ATI indicated whether there was a matching effect in the hypothesized direction over the entire test period (e.g., months 4–15). There were also two indicators of whether the ATI effect changed significantly over time: an ATI by linear time effect, and an ATI by quadratic time effect. Analyses involving these time effects were centered at the midpoint of the test period. Because time contrasts were not directional, significant interactions related to time were tested on a month-by-month basis to determine how they were changing over time.

Successful treatment matching is not, however, precisely synonymous with an interaction effect. A hypothesis test for a matching attribute by treatment interaction simply indicates whether the difference between two treatments is the same for all values of the matching variable. It is theoretically possible for a significant ATI to occur when one treatment is superior to the other for all values of the matching variable (commonly called an ordinal interaction, see Chapter 1). Thus, a significant ATI is a necessary, but not a sufficient, condition for matching to occur in the sense that recommendations about clinical outcomes would vary according to the level of the matching variable. Any significant ATI found in Project MATCH was therefore followed by additional *post hoc* tests to determine its clinical significance. Additional analyses were also conducted to test the theory underlying each *a priori* matching hypothesis (i.e., the hypothesized causal chain).

Missing data

The primary analyses followed an approach that included all randomized clients, regardless of the degree to which they participated in treatment. Thus, participants who failed to attend any, and those who completed very few, of the recommended therapy sessions were included in the analyses if they had sufficient follow-up data. Clients were included in the analyses if they had non-missing data for at least two-thirds of the time points in the test period. As detailed in Chapter 5, follow-up participation rates were quite high (ranging from 92% to 98% for the five sessions conducted during the post-treatment period), and rates did not differ as a function of treatment condition. As a consequence, missing data rates were very low: roughly 7% of Outpatient clients had to be dropped from post-treatment analyses because of missing outcome data. A small number of additional participants were excluded from some matching tests because of missing data on the matching attribute in the analysis. Ancillary analyses indicated that the primary analysis results were not sensitive to missing data exclusion. (See Project MATCH Research Group, 1997a, for additional information regarding missing data.)

Three-year follow-up analyses

Rather than trying to extend the latent growth model used in analyses of months 1–3 and 4–15 well beyond the point at which quadratic latent growth curves might be acceptable, the 3-year follow-up data were analyzed separately. Because there were no significant time trends for drinking measures summed across each month in the 90-day assessment window evaluated at follow-up (months 37–39), outcome data were aggregated across the period and summary measures of PDA and DDD were used as the dependent measure in an analysis of covariance. The covariates were baseline drinking, CRU main effects, and CRU by treatment interactions.

Three-year follow-up data were obtained from 85% of the original Outpatient sample, and there were no statistically significant differences across treatments in follow-up rate. Of the missing participants, approximately 5% could not be located, 8% refused to be interviewed, and 3% were known to have died. Missing data analyses indicated that the 806 participants who completed the long-term follow-up interview did not differ from the 146 missing cases on baseline values of either of the two primary drinking measures (PDA, DDD), basic demographic variables, or many of the primary or secondary matching attribute variables. Thus, the assessed cases were found to be representative of the original Outpatient sample. (See Project MATCH Research Group, 1998a, for more details regarding the 3-year follow-up data analytic procedures.)

Results

Although separate analyses were conducted for each major phase of the trial, the results of the analyses of the primary drinking outcomes are organized and presented in terms of specific effects in order to show the continuities and discontinuities of the findings across time. Effects for time, site, treatment condition, and prognostic factors are presented first, followed by a description of treatment matching results.

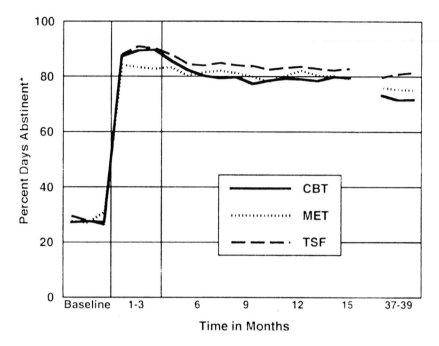

Percent Days Abstinent by Treatment Condition

* Estimated from transformed data

Figure 7.3 Monthly Percent Days Abstinent (PDA) for Outpatient clients
assigned to Cognitive–Behavioral Therapy (CBT), Motivational Enhancement
Therapy (MET) and Twelve Step Facilitation therapy (TSF) for baseline
(averaged over 3 months prior to treatment), within treatment (months 1–3), the
year following treatment (months 4–15), and (after a 2-year gap) the long-term
follow-up period (months 37–39). (Adapted from Project MATCH Research
Group, 1997a.)

Trends over time

Figures 7.3 and 7.4 summarize the main findings in relation to treatment
effects and changes in drinking over time. The baseline period shown in
each of the two figures represents a 90-day period prior to enrollment in
the trial. In general, there were large, statistically significant reductions in
drinking between baseline and each of the follow-up points, but only

Drinks per Drinking Day by Treatment Condition

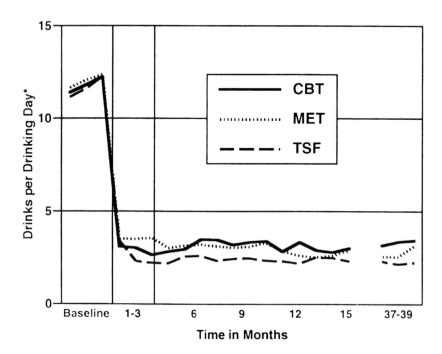

* Estimated from transformed data

Figure 7.4 Monthly Drinks per Drinking Day (DDD) for Outpatient clients assigned to Cognitive–Behavioral Therapy (CBT), Motivational Enhancement Therapy (MET) and Twelve Step Facilitation therapy (TSF), for baseline (averaged over 3 months prior to treatment), within treatment (months 1–3), the year following treatment (months 4–15), and (after a 2-year gap) the long-term follow-up period (months 37–39). (Adapted from Project MATCH Research Group, 1997a.)

minimal differences among the three treatment groups. As shown in the figures, PDA and DDD levels improved substantially from baseline to the end of treatment, and overall levels of drinking increased only slightly across months 4–15. As shown in Figure 7.3, the frequency of abstinent days changed from roughly 30% at baseline to more than 80% at post-treatment, with only a slight decrement at the 15-month follow-up point.

Dramatic improvements were also evident for DDD (Fig. 7.4), with drinks per day declining from approximately 13 at pre-treatment to about three during the follow-up phase. There were also significant CRU main effects for both dependent variables during the post-treatment period, but not during the 12 weeks of active treatment, indicating that the prognosis for clients at different sites varied across the 1-year follow-up period. These effects were partly, but not wholly, accounted for by baseline differences in drinking severity.

The reductions in drinking that were observed in the first year after treatment were generally sustained at the 3-year follow-up point. Almost 30% of the subjects were totally abstinent in months 37–39, and the median value for PDA for those who did report drinking was 68%.

Treatment effects

During the phase of active treatment (months 1–3), small but statistically significant differences among treatments were found for the PDA outcome, with clients in Cognitive–Behavioral Coping Skills Therapy (CBT) and Twelve Step Facilitation (TSF) consuming alcohol less frequently (on average, 2 days less per month) than those in Motivational Enhancement Therapy (MET). There was also a significant treatment by linear time interaction for DDD. Beginning at week 9, clients in CBT consumed, on average, one drink less per drinking day than their counterparts in MET. One possible reason for this effect, which faded during the post-treatment follow-up period, lies in the intensity difference between MET and the other therapies (four versus 12 sessions). This interpretation is supported by the finding that differences in drinking intensity emerged late in the treatment phase, when the differences in treatment intensity were greatest.

In addition to these effects, significant CRU by treatment interactions indicated that the relative effectiveness of the three treatments varied across the Outpatient sites. Analyses were conducted to explore whether these effects were due to variations across sites in the implementation of the Project MATCH interventions. These analyses failed to reveal any substantial, clinically meaningful differences in treatment implementation variables (e.g., therapist skillfulness, therapeutic alliance). In the light of these interactions, however, we cannot conclude that there were any generalizable treatment main effects for either of the two drinking outcome measures (Project MATCH Research Group, 1998a).

For the post-treatment follow-up period (months 4–15) there were no overall treatment main effects for either of the two drinking outcome measures, although there were small and statistically significant treatment by time interactions. However, significant CRU by treatment effects for both PDA and DDD indicated that treatment efficacy varied widely from site to site. These effects, coupled with the small magnitude and shifting temporal pattern of the overall treatment effects, suggest that there were no consistent and clinically meaningful differences in the efficacy of the three treatments (Project MATCH Research Group, 1997a).

CRU by treatment interactions, which had been present at earlier time points, were not detected at the 3-year follow-up. As in the earlier periods, there were few differences among the three treatments, although TSF did show an advantage over CBT in some analyses (Project MATCH Research Group, 1998b).

Prognostic effects

Table 7.1 lists the client attributes designated in the *a priori* primary and secondary treatment matching hypotheses. As described more fully in the preceding chapter, those characteristics judged to have the strongest empirical evidence, or the most compelling theoretical rationale, were labeled as *primary a priori* matching variables. Those that appeared promising to the investigators, but had less empirical support or weaker theoretical justification, were designated as *secondary a priori* matching variables. In addition to treatment main effects and interaction effects, the main effects of the matching variables themselves were examined in the analyses. Table 7.1 indicates which of these client attributes produced significant main effects (unqualified by time) on treatment outcomes during the 1-year follow-up period and, later, at the 3-year follow-up point.

As shown in the table, seven of the 21 variables had prognostic effects during the 1-year post-treatment period, and 11 were predictive of drinking outcomes at the 3-year follow-up. The most consistent predictors were Motivation and Readiness to Change. These conceptually related variables were significantly related to both PDA and DDD in both time frames. The two Self-efficacy measures were also associated with treatment outcomes across the two time periods. Although effects were found for both dependent measures, the effect of Support for Drinking was limited to the 1-year post-treatment phase. Indicators of the severity of alcohol-related problems – Alcohol Involvement, Typology, and Alcohol

Dependence – exerted effects on long-term drinking outcomes. Other effects were more limited in terms of time or outcome measure.

In summary, during the 12 months following the end of treatment (months 4–15), the best pre-treatment predictors of future abstinence were higher levels of Motivation, lower Support for Drinking, greater severity of Alcohol Dependence, and higher Self-efficacy and Readiness to Change. Conversely, when relapse occurred, higher levels of consumption (DDD) were predicted by lower pre-treatment Motivation and Readiness to Change, more Support for Drinking, and lower scores on Religiosity, and Self-efficacy. At the 3-year follow-up point, abstinence was associated with greater pre-treatment Alcohol Involvement, Meaning Seeking, Motivation, Type B alcoholism (high vulnerability, high severity), more severe Alcohol Dependence, Prior Engagement in Alcoholics Anonymous (AA), poorer Social Functioning, and higher Readiness to Change. Conversely, the strongest predictors of drinking intensity (DDD) at the 3-year follow-up were lower Alcohol Involvement, Motivation, Religiosity, Self-efficacy, and Readiness to Change.

Tests of matching hypotheses

Results of tests of the 21 primary and secondary *a priori* client–treatment matching hypotheses are summarized in Table 7.2. As shown in the table, few hypotheses were statistically supported and, for those that were significant, the results were generally inconsistent across time and outcome measure.

Hypothesis tests failed to find any interaction effects that had an impact on drinking throughout the 12-week treatment phase, i.e., an ATI that did not interact with time. One primary matching hypothesis, Support for Drinking, yielded significant attribute by treatment by time effects for both drinking outcome measures during the early weeks of treatment. This hypothesis predicted that clients with higher social network support for drinking would fare better in TSF than in MET. (A parallel hypothesis involving CBT and MET was not supported.) Weekly contrasts showed that this interaction effect was significant during the first 3 weeks of therapy for PDA and during the first 4 weeks for DDD.

As indicated in Table 7.2, the Support for Drinking hypothesis was not confirmed in analyses of the 1-year post-treatment data. However, significant matching effects did emerge for both drinking outcome measures at the 3-year follow-up. These results are presented in Figure 7.5, which

Table 7.1. *Significant prognostic effects of primary and secondary matching attributes on primary drinking outcomes*[a]

	Post-treatment (months 4–15)		Three-year follow-up	
	Percent Days Abstinent	Drinks per Drinking Day	Percent Days Abstinent	Drinks per Drinking Day
Primary matching variable				
Alcohol Involvement			+	−
Cognitive Impairment				
Conceptual Level				
Gender				
Meaning Seeking			+	
Motivation	+	−	+	−
Psychiatric Severity				
Support for Drinking	−	+		
Sociopathy				
Typology			+	
Secondary matching variable				
Alcohol Dependence	+		+	
Anger				
Antisocial Personality Disorder				
Interpersonal Dependency				
Psychopathology DSM-III-R Axis I Diagnosis				
Prior Engagement in AA	+		+	
Readiness to Change		−	+	−
Religiosity		−		−

Self-efficacy			
Confidence	+	−	−
Temptation minus Confidence	−	+	+
Social Functioning		−	

[a]Only main (non-time-dependent) effects are shown. Entries indicate the direction of the prognostic main effect with a blank space, indicating no significant effect in that category. Additional details regarding the nature of the effects listed in this table can be found in primary sources (Project MATCH Research Group, 1997a; 1997b; 1998a).

Table 7.2. *Statistically significant treatment matching effects across time*

Matching hypothesis	Treatment contrast	Drinking outcome	Within-treatment effect	Post-treatment (4–15 months) effect	Three-year follow-up effect
Primary matching variable					
Conceptual Level	TSF vs. MET	DDD		ATI[a] × time	
Motivation	MET vs. CBT	PDA		ATI × time	
Psychiatric Severity	CBT vs. TSF	PDA		ATI, ATI × time	
Support for Drinking	TSF vs. MET	PDA	ATI × time		ATI
		DDD	ATI × time		ATI
Secondary matching variable					
Anger	MET vs. (CBT & TSF)	PDA		ATI	ATI
		DDD		ATI	ATI
Antisocial Personality Disorder	MET vs. TSF	PDA		ATI × time	
		DDD	ATI × time		

[a] ATI = attribute × treatment interaction. See text for details regarding methods of analysis. Additional details regarding the nature of the effects listed in this table can be found in primary sources (Project MATCH Research Group, 1997a; 1997b; 1998a; 1998b). CBT, Cognitive–Behavioral Therapy; TSF, Twelve Step Facilitation; MET, Motivational Enhancement Therapy; PDA, Percent Days Abstinent; DDD, Drinks per Drinking Day.

Social Support for Drinking Matching Effect at 3 Years

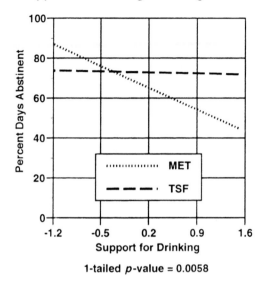

1-tailed *p*-value = 0.0058

1-tailed *p*-value = 0.0035

Figure 7.5 Social Support for Drinking matching effect at 3 years, Motivational Enhancement Therapy (MET) versus Twelve Step Facilitation therapy (TSF) contrast on two primary outcome measures, Percent Days Abstinent (PDA) and Drinks per Drinking Day (DDD). (Adapted from Longabaugh et al., 1998.)

shows that clients whose social networks were more supportive of drinking derived greater benefit from TSF than from MET. Among clients in the highest third of the Support for Drinking measure, those in TSF were abstinent 16.3% more days than those in MET. At the lower end of this variable, the difference in PDA between MET and TSF was 3.8%, with MET clients having more abstinent days. For the DDD measure, TSF clients in the upper third drank 1.5 fewer drinks per drinking day than those in MET, whereas for clients in the lower third this difference was 1.1 drinks, favoring those in MET (Project MATCH Research Group, 1998a).

The secondary hypothesis Antisocial Personality Disorder (ASPD) also achieved significance in the analysis of the within-treatment period, but the effect was limited to the last 2 weeks of therapy. During this limited time window, TSF clients with an ASPD diagnosis consumed fewer drinks per drinking day than those in MET. A significant time-dependent effect was obtained for PDA in the analyses of the 1-year post-treatment time frame. However, the change over time was so small that it did not involve a significant effect in any single month of the period.

In the year following the end of treatment (months 4–15), significant matching effects emerged for three of the *a priori* primary matching hypotheses: Conceptual Level, Motivation, and Psychiatric Severity. However, for Conceptual Level, none of the monthly tests of the hypothesized contrast approached a 0.05 level of statistical significance.

A significant ATI by time effect was detected for Motivation. Immediately after treatment (month 4), CBT clients low in Motivation were found to have better outcomes than their counterparts in MET. However, this trend is the opposite of what had been predicted. By month 15, the matching effect reversed, so that, relative to CBT, MET produced superior outcomes for low Motivation cases. This time-varying effect, in combination with the strong prognostic effects for Motivation, suggested that a Motivation matching effect might again be found at the 3-year follow-up point. However, as indicated in Table 7.2, the matching effect was not maintained.

The matching effect for Psychiatric Severity, as measured by the Addiction Severity Index (ASI), was also found to vary in magnitude over time (a significant Psychiatric Severity by treatment by time interaction). However, it was strong enough across the bulk of the outcome period to attain overall statistical significance. The pattern of this matching effect over time is shown in Figure 7.6. As indicated in the figure, starting in month 4, people low in Psychiatric Severity had superior outcomes when treated in

Psychiatric Severity Matching Effect Over Time

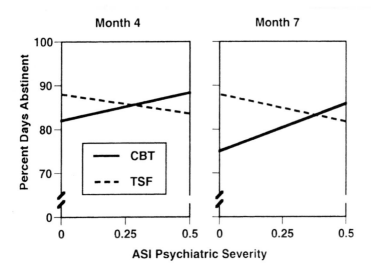

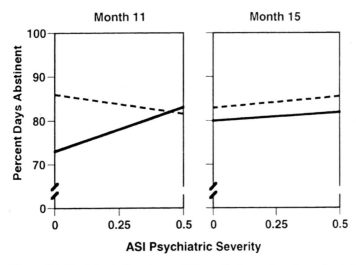

Figure 7.6 Psychiatric Severity matching effect over time (months 4, 7, 11, and 15) showing treatment by time by attribute interaction for Psychiatric Severity contrast between Cognitive–Behavioral Therapy (CBT) and Twelve Step Facilitation therapy (TSF). The vertical axis represents Percent Days Abstinent (PDA) and the horizontal axis represents Addiction Severity Index (ASI) Psychiatric Severity scores. (Adapted from Project MATCH Research Group, 1997a.)

TSF rather than in CBT. The matching effect was significant from month 5 through 11, after which it waned and disappeared by month 15. At higher levels of Psychiatric Severity, there may be some superiority of CBT over TSF. However, there were too few cases high enough in Psychiatric Severity to demonstrate this effect conclusively. Moreover, the effect was not significant at the 3-year follow-up.

As already noted, post-treatment tests of the secondary matching hypotheses produced significant results for ASPD. In addition, the matching hypothesis involving Anger also received strong support: significant effects were found for both PDA and DDD in both the 1-year and 3-year analyses (see Fig. 7.7). As predicted, MET clients with higher levels of Anger had a higher frequency of abstinent days, and lower quantities of consumption per drinking occasion, than those in TSF and in CBT. At the 3-year follow-up point, MET participants in the highest third on the Anger variable had, on average, 76% abstinent days, while their counterparts in the other two treatments (CBT and TSF) had, on average, 66% abstinent days. Conversely, clients low in Anger performed better after treatment in CBT and in TSF than in MET. The same pattern was found for DDD: MET clients with higher Anger scores reported 4.9 drinks per drinking day, compared to 6.3 for those in the other two treatment conditions, whereas participants with lower levels of Anger fared better in CBT and in TSF than in MET (Project MATCH Research Group, 1998a).

Two additional findings emerged from the post-treatment analyses. Both the Social Functioning and Typology matching variables produced effects opposite to what was predicted. It had been hypothesized that poor Social Functioning would be associated with more favorable outcomes in CBT than in MET or in TSF. Instead, relative to MET and TSF, higher functioning clients in CBT had a greater proportion of abstinent days and consumed fewer drinks per drinking day during both the within-treatment and follow-up periods. The Typology variable, which partitioned clients into two groups on the basis of a cluster of interrelated factors reflecting premorbid vulnerability and current problem severity, also had a significant effect opposite from the original prediction in the 3-year analyses. As described more fully in Chapter 6, relative to Type A clients (low vulnerability, low severity), Type B participants (high vulnerability, high severity) in CBT and TSF were expected to have more favorable outcomes than those in MET, but this did not occur.

This section describes the results of Project MATCH in relation to the primary purpose of the study, i.e., the evaluation of client–treatment

Anger Matching Effect at 3 Years

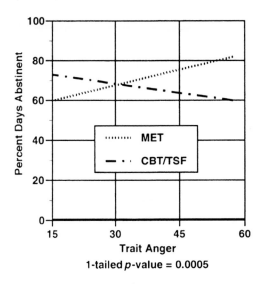

1-tailed *p*-value = 0.0005

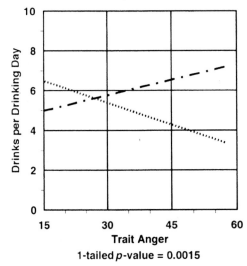

1-tailed *p*-value = 0.0015

Figure 7.7 Anger matching effect at 3-year follow-up point for Cognitive–
Behavioral Therapy/Twelve Step Facilitation (CBT/TSF) and Motivational
Enhancement Therapy (MET). (Adapted from Project MATCH Research
Group, 1998a.)

matching. Despite the theoretical and empirical rationale marshaled for the 21 *a priori* hypotheses, only three – Psychiatric Severity, Support for Drinking, and Anger – received support in the analyses of the Outpatient sample, and only one of the three – Anger – produced a significant effect for both outcome variables that was robust across time. Thus, the results do not offer compelling support for the general hypothesis that drinking outcomes can be markedly improved by triaging clients to one or another of the three study treatments on the basis of individual characteristics.

Exploratory analyses

Although 21 potential matching variables were included in the *a priori* analyses, it was still possible that other variables might produce matching effects, or that the *a priori* variables could have unexpected kinds of matching effects. To study these possibilities, exploratory matching analyses were conducted using a simplified analytical method. PDA and DDD for months 4–15 were averaged across months, and these summary scores were used in regression analyses. In addition to the 21 *a priori* matching attributes, 20 variables (Table 7.3) were used as predictors in a forward step-wise regression analysis performed within each treatment condition. In these analyses, the pre-treatment value of the dependent variable and treatment site (CRU) were entered first, followed by the remaining variables in a forward step-wise manner. A variable having significant effects within any one treatment condition was included in additional analyses if the size or sign of its *beta* coefficients varied across treatments. In final hierarchical regression analyses, variables were entered in the following order: simple effects for baseline drinking, CRU, and the potential matching variable; two-way interaction terms involving the matching attribute, CRU, and treatment; and the three-way interaction between attribute, CRU, and treatment. An ATI was considered statistically significant if it met the $p < 0.05$ *alpha* criterion, and there was no significant three-way interaction term. This same strategy was repeated using a second set of potential matching variables, the 15 primary subscales (excluding marital scales) from the Alcohol Use Inventory (AUI: Horn et al., 1990), as predictor variables.

To control for a Type I error in the exploratory analyses, a random sample comprised of two-thirds of the Outpatient participants was selected for the main set of exploratory analyses, and the remaining one-third of the

Table 7.3. *Client attributes tested in exploratory treatment matching analyses*

Demographic characteristics
Age
Years of education
Marital status
Occupational prestige
Years at current address
Number of paid work days[a]

Alcohol-related measures
Percent Days Abstinent[a]
Drinks per Drinking Day[a]
Age of first drinking problem
Days since last drink
Number of illegal drugs used
Number of prior alcohol treatment episodes
MacAndrew Alcoholism Scale of the Minnesota Multiphasic Personality
    Inventory (MMPI)
Coercion into treatment[b]
Family history of alcohol problems (Addiction Severity Index, ASI)

Psychological variables
Beck Depression Inventory score
Control versus Impulse Subscale of the Differential Personality Questionnaire
History of lifetime physical/emotional/sexual abuse (ASI)

Social functioning
Social support from family
Social support from friends

---

[a]Based on a 90-day pre-treatment time window.
[b]Based on responses to two questions: 'Was seeking treatment prompted by the criminal justice system?' (ASI) and 'Have others "pushed" you to take treatment for a drinking problem?' (Alcohol Use Inventory, AUI).

sample was used for replicating the results. An interaction was considered reliable if it was found to replicate on the holdout sample.

Under these conditions, only one variable, Social Functioning, was found to interact with treatment in the initial round of exploratory analyses, and this was only for the PDA outcome measure. As in the analyses of the secondary matching hypotheses, this interaction effect was opposite to what was originally predicted. That is, higher functioning clients in CBT had more favorable outcomes than their counterparts in MET and TSF. Moreover, the effect size was small and did not replicate in the holdout sample. To summarize, we found little support for additional client–treatment matches beyond those variables selected for *a priori* study.

Causal chain analyses and clinical significance of matching

As part of the trial's *a priori* analysis plan, the research team associated with each of the primary and secondary hypotheses was required to develop a theoretical rationale that specified the causal chain underlying the predictions that were made (see Chapter 6). Analyses testing the linkages in these causal chains were conducted for each matching attribute, regardless of whether or not the hypothesis was empirically supported. For hypotheses that were supported, investigators examined different aspects of the therapy process and other intermediate variables to determine whether the observed matching effects were attributable to the postulated mechanisms. More detail regarding the causal chain analyses for these and the other *a priori* matching hypotheses can be found in Longabaugh and Wirtz (2001).

In addition to the causal chain analyses, the potential clinical importance of each statistically significant matching result was examined by comparing the outcomes of participants who had been matched to treatment with those who had been mismatched according to the hypothesis specifications. At each follow-up time point, clients were classified as treatment 'successes' or 'failures' based upon their Composite outcome category assignments (see Chapter 3). An outcome was deemed a success if the client was either abstinent or drinking moderately and not experiencing alcohol-related problems; the outcome was classified as a 'failure' if the participant reported any heavy drinking and/or negative consequences during the 3-month assessment period. For each matching attribute, a cut-off score was used to partition clients into 'low' and 'high' scoring groups and, for each hypothesized treatment contrast, success and failure outcomes were examined for clients designated as 'matched,' 'mismatched,' or 'nonmatched' to treatment. To assess the relative advantage of matching clients to treatments, the outcomes for these groups were evaluated relative to those of *all* clients who had been assigned to the specific treatments that were contrasted in the matching hypothesis. In the following sections, the causal chain results and the clinical significance of matching are described for the three matching hypotheses that were supported in the Outpatient study analyses: Psychiatric Severity, Anger, and Support for Drinking.

Psychiatric Severity

According to the Psychiatric Severity matching hypothesis, CBT, unlike the other therapies, had specific components designed to manage the psychiatric conditions often associated with alcoholism. Whereas TSF and MET had been developed uniquely for the treatment of alcoholism, CBT was viewed as a more general approach, because it had been used extensively in the treatment of anxiety and depression. Thus, it was predicted that CBT would address the problems of clients with high Psychiatric Severity scores better than the other interventions, and that ultimately drinking outcomes would reflect the attention directed at this specific risk factor for relapse.

Analyses provided only partial support for the hypothesized causal chain. As noted previously, relatively few clients had high levels of psychopathology. Analyses examining the treatment experiences of this subset of clients suggested that there were few differences among therapies in terms of their attention to psychopathology symptoms. Also, although psychopathology evidenced at the end of treatment was linked to subsequent drinking, there was no evidence to indicate that CBT was more successful in reducing symptoms than TSF or MET. Both CBT and TSF were associated with decreased psychopathology, perhaps secondary to reductions in alcohol consumption (Cooney et al., 2001).

The clinical implications of the Psychiatric Severity results were further explored in terms of the relative proportions of treatment successes and failures observed for matched participants and those in other comparison groups. Clients were divided into low and high psychopathology groups on the basis of their ASI Psychiatric Severity scores. High psychopathology clients were considered to be matched to treatment when randomly assigned to CBT and mismatched when assigned to TSF. Conversely, low psychopathology participants were regarded as matched in TSF and mismatched in CBT. A small matching effect was evident during treatment; this effect endured through month 11 (i.e., 9 months following the end of treatment). Matched clients had approximately a 5% higher success rate than mismatched clients. It appears that only a minority of clients would benefit materially from matching.

Anger

Although the Anger hypothesis received relatively strong empirical support, attempts to confirm the predicted mechanism underlying the effect
were generally not successful. According to the hypothesis formulation,
participants with higher Anger scores were expected to be more resistant to
treatment than their less angry counterparts and to benefit differentially
from MET because this treatment is designed to mollify resistance and
mobilize the client's own resources in the service of recovery. The first step
in the causal chain analyses therefore investigated the relationship between
Anger and resistance, which was operationalized in terms of two of the
SOCRATES subscales, Problem Recognition and Taking Steps Toward
Change. Contrary to predictions, the matching attribute was not substantially correlated with the two scale scores. Further analyses focused on
how Anger might influence the process of therapy. Three measures derived
from the Working Alliance Inventory – Therapeutic Bond, Goal Agreement, and Task Agreement – were investigated in relation to client Anger
and treatment outcome. Contrary to the predicted causal chain, process
measures did not mediate the observed matching effect. However, resistance was an important variable within the matching effect (see Waldron et
al., 2001). Thus, despite the strong evidence for treatment matching, the
causal chain analyses indicate that the mechanisms underlying the effect
are not fully understood. Whether this lack of understanding is a product
of methodological limitations or a result of incorrect theoretical specification is unclear.

Outcome comparisons indicated that clients who were matched on the
basis of the Anger hypothesis had approximately a 10% higher success rate
than mismatched clients, and roughly a 5% higher success rate than
nonmatched participants. However, in the first 6 months after treatment,
all participants assigned to TSF (regardless of their Anger scores) had
outcomes as good as those for matched clients. Using the 'success' criteria
of either abstinence or moderate drinking without problems, a treatment
main effect favoring TSF was evident early in the follow-up year. This
effect diminished later in the post-treatment follow-up period, and the
Anger effect became dominant.

Support for Drinking

The Support for Drinking hypothesis predicted that clients whose social
networks were supportive of alcohol use would fare better in either CBT or

TSF than in MET. CBT was thought to be conducive to improved outcomes because it would teach skills for coping with others who were supportive of drinking. TSF was expected to encourage involvement in AA, which would provide social support for abstinence. MET, on the other hand, was viewed as lacking any mechanism for reducing vulnerability to social network support for drinking. As indicated above, a significant matching result was obtained for the MET versus TSF contrast (but not the CBT contrast) for both primary drinking outcomes (PDA and DDD) at the 3-year follow-up point.

Unlike the other matching hypotheses, the causal chain analyses for the Support for Drinking effect provided some support for the theory underlying the prediction. As hypothesized, AA involvement was a partial mediator of the matching effect. TSF clients with social networks that were supportive of drinking were more likely to participate in AA. High AA involvement (averaged over the 1-year post-treatment follow-up period) was evident for 62% of these clients compared with 38% of those in MET and 25% in CBT. To complete the causal chain, AA involvement was associated with better drinking outcomes (higher PDA and fewer DDD) 3 years post-treatment for TSF clients with social networks that were highly supportive of drinking at the start of the trial (Longabaugh et al., 1998).

The matching effect was also evaluated in terms of the treatment success versus failure measure. For this comparison, clients with social networks that were strongly supportive of drinking were considered matched when they were randomly assigned to TSF, and mismatched when assigned to MET. Participants with low network support for drinking were regarded as matched in MET and mismatched in TSF. The results indicated a small matching effect during the treatment phase (corresponding to the time-dependent ATI noted above). This effect diminished during the year after treatment, and it re-emerged at the 3-year follow-up point. Matched clients had a success rate 7% higher than mismatched participants, and 3% higher than those who were assigned randomly during the treatment phase and, again, 3 years following the end of treatment.

Discussion

Perhaps the most notable finding from the analyses of the Outpatient sample is the considerable reductions in the frequency and intensity of drinking that followed enrollment in Project MATCH, decreases that were largely sustained at the 3-year follow-up point. Rather than gradually taking effect as treatment progresses, these changes are most pronounced at the beginning of treatment, and the improvements evident at the end of treatment show only modest declines over the course of the follow-up period. The stability of group average outcomes, however, should not be taken to imply that individual outcomes show the same pattern. Indeed, other analyses show that, while there is significant overlap between the individuals who are successful at one point and those who are successful at another, there are also numerous instances where an apparent failure at one point shines out as a success at some later time. Analyses of prognostic variables may help us to understand better the processes associated with good long-term outcome. The group average findings reported here should not be construed to suggest that all participants improved at the same rate. As shown in Chapter 9, other outcome measures indicate substantial variability in drinking patterns, with some clients achieving complete abstinence and others demonstrating continued problem drinking.

Although substantial declines in drinking were observed across the various phases of the trial, there were few indications in analyses of the primary drinking outcome measures that any one of the three treatments was superior to the others. Further, this general lack of differences between treatments seems not to be attributable to the effects of matching or mismatching clients to therapy on the basis of personal attributes. Tests of 21 *a priori* matching hypotheses, supplemented by exploratory analyses involving an additional 34 participant characteristics (including the 15 AUI subscales), failed to produce robust matching results. Further, the clinical implications of the matching effects that were obtained are not entirely clear. Although clients matched to treatment (*post hoc*, on the basis of the significant matching hypotheses) fared better than those who were mismatched, the differentials tended to be relatively small. Although results may vary depending upon the criteria used to define treatment success and failure, the bulk of the evidence suggests that the 'value added' to treatment outcome by matching on the basis of client attributes is not great.

It is noteworthy that most, although not all, of the major effects detected in the Outpatient arm varied over time, within as well as across the three analytical periods. The effects detected during the active treatment phase did not carry over after treatment ended, and most of the effects seen in the first year after treatment were not maintained 3 years later. The Anger matching effect is a notable exception; while not present during treatment, it nonetheless persisted throughout months 4 through 15 and extended to the 3-year follow-up point.

One obvious implication of the findings is the need to understand recovery as a process with multiple phases. From one perspective, this is discouraging in that there are relatively few simple lessons to derive from the Project MATCH results. From another perspective, however, we can see from these data that the period around the beginning of treatment is one when rapid change is often taking place. Treatment may affect some, but not all, of those changes, and may also alter the path of change so that some long-term impacts can persist or even emerge after a delay.

One of the general conclusions from the causal chain analyses is that many of the postulated differential treatment effects failed to materialize. Although the treatments were highly discriminable (see Chapter 4), the differences between the treatments failed in the majority of instances to generate the predicted differential effects on critical mediating variables. The exceptions are the evidence for the Support for Drinking causal chain and the partial confirmation of the mediational path for the Anger hypothesis.

Because alcoholism is a chronic, relapsing disorder whose course is typically measured in years, the two matching effects observed at the 3-year follow-up deserve close attention. Both are true matching effects; that is, they imply different treatment recommendations depending on the level of the client attribute. The Anger matching results suggest the importance of engagement in treatment. Whereas the predicted differential therapy processes did not occur during the treatment phase, a difficult first course of treatment may set the stage for problems later. The processes underlying the Anger matching effect will require further study. The late-emerging Support for Drinking matching effect suggests that changes in social network mechanisms may be important for sustained long-term improvement for many clients who live in social environments that encourage drinking. Although the magnitude of the matching effect is relatively small when considered in terms of the treatment success criterion used to investigate clinical significance, the causal chain analyses did provide some support for the theory underlying the effect. The mechanisms that underlie this matching effect, however, will require careful consideration if treatments optimally capable of producing this effect are to be designed. Further exploration of these findings in relation to AA affiliation is presented in Chapter 11.

The significance of the ASI Psychiatric Severity matching effect is somewhat undermined by its time-limited nature. Nonetheless, it deserves further study because even modest increments in treatment effectiveness via matching are difficult to find. Furthermore, the fact that the matching effect was found across a period of several months suggests that it may be possible to adjust treatment protocols to extend the time and enlarge the effect. We can only speculate that the limited duration of the matching effect might be due to resolution over that time period of the psychiatric impairment indicated by the baseline ASI Psychiatric Severity score. Further research is also needed into the treatment of clients who present with higher levels of psychiatric impairment than was typical of Project MATCH participants.

Finally, the sustained level of outcome seen across months 4–15 and again at the 3-year follow-up point is clear evidence that alcoholism is a treatable disorder whose long-term course is not necessarily one of uniform deterioration. Although some study participants at 3 years showed high levels of drinking and poor functional outcomes, many were substantially improved relative to their pre-treatment status.

8

Primary treatment outcomes and matching effects: Aftercare arm

CARRIE L. RANDALL, FRANCES K. DEL BOCA,
MARGARET E. MATTSON, ROBERT RYCHTARIK, NED L. COONEY,
DENNIS M. DONOVAN, RICHARD LONGABAUGH,
AND PHILIP W. WIRTZ

Residential and day-hospital rehabilitation programs play an important role in the treatment of people with alcohol dependence, particularly those with more severe and persistent problems. This chapter describes the results for the Aftercare arm of Project MATCH, which investigated treatment matching in clients who had just completed a program of conventional inpatient or day-hospital treatment. As with the Outpatient arm, there was no evidence for the superiority of any one treatment over another on the primary drinking outcome measures, and clients improved significantly from baseline through the 15-month follow-up period, both in the frequency and in the intensity of drinking. With regard to matching effects, only one of the 21 *a priori* matching hypotheses was confirmed. Clients with more severe alcohol dependence had better post-treatment outcomes in Twelve Step Facilitation therapy, whereas lower scoring participants fared better in Cognitive–Behavioral Therapy. The clinical significance of this matching effect is discussed, and the results of the Outpatient and Aftercare arms of the study are compared.

Residential rehabilitation programs had become the standard of care for alcoholism treatment in the USA by the late 1980s. It is therefore not surprising that, prior to Project MATCH, treatment matching research in alcoholics primarily utilized clients who were enrolled in, or had recently completed, traditional inpatient treatment programs (Mattson et al., 1994). The *a priori* matching hypotheses described in Chapter 6 were based upon such research, where positive results of treatment matching had been suggested in single-site studies (Project MATCH Research Group, 1993; Mattson et al., 1994). This chapter reports results for the Aftercare arm of Project MATCH, which investigated treatment matching in clients who had already completed a program of conventional inpatient treatment. This component of the trial was used to test matching hypotheses within what was the dominant treatment context at the time the trial began, and it did so using a participant sample which was quite similar to those in earlier studies with promising matching results.

This chapter begins with a description of the Aftercare Clinical Research Units (CRUs) and the treatment programs that served as recruitment sites. Next, treatment effects and matching results are reported for the trial's two primary drinking outcome measures. Findings for additional secondary outcome measures are reported in Chapter 9. Results are presented for both the primary and secondary *a priori* treatment matching hypotheses and for a set of exploratory analyses aimed at uncovering any unanticipated matching results. Next, causal chain analyses are summarized for the one hypothesis that was supported empirically. The chapter concludes by comparing the results for the Aftercare arm of the trial with those presented in the preceding chapter for the Outpatient study.

Method

Recruitment sites

Initially, there were four Aftercare CRUs located in Charleston, South Carolina; Houston, Texas; Providence, Rhode Island; and Seattle, Washington. As third-party payers began to limit reimbursement for conventional inpatient treatment programs, a fifth CRU, located in Milwaukee, Wisconsin, was added to increase the pace of recruitment. To meet enrollment objectives, all five of the Aftercare CRUs recruited clients from multiple inpatient programs. For three sites (Charleston, Houston, and Seattle), local Veterans Administration (VA) hospitals served as the major recruitment source, and VA patients comprised 40% of the Aftercare sample. The Providence CRU recruited primarily from a private hospital, and the Milwaukee site enrolled patients from treatment centers affiliated with the local Health Maintenance Organization. Over the course of the 2-year enrollment period (from 1991 to 1993), 774 clients were recruited from 27 different programs.

At the time that the trial began, most inpatient recruitment facilities operated traditional 21-day or 28-day treatment programs. As the trial progressed, the length of stay decreased markedly at all recruitment sites, and some inpatient programs closed. To be eligible for participation, prospective clients had to have completed a program that was at least 7 days in length and that offered some type of therapeutic service beyond medical detoxification. One site, Providence, enrolled patients from a day-hospital program. All other CRUs recruited from traditional in-patient programs that required overnight stays. Length of stay varied from 7 to 44 days, with an average of 21 days.

The inpatient treatment programs at all recruitment sites delivered traditional, Alcoholics Anonymous (AA)-oriented treatment with group therapy, family counseling, and educational groups. AA meeting attendance was mandatory at most facilities. The staffing was typically multidisciplinary, including physicians, psychologists, social workers, nurses, and counselors. Aftercare clients were recruited directly from the various inpatient treatment programs, and enrollment typically occurred during the final week of treatment. Whenever possible, baseline assessments and the first Project MATCH treatment session were conducted prior to discharge. When length of stay became shorter, clients were recruited soon after admission.

Clients who appeared to meet the Aftercare eligibility criteria were asked about their interest in participating in Project MATCH and their willingness to accept random assignment to aftercare treatment. With the exception of the inpatient treatment requirement, inclusion/exclusion criteria and assessment procedures for the Aftercare arm of the trial were the same as those for the Outpatient study.

Research participants

As described more fully in Chapter 5, the 774 Aftercare participants were broadly representative of the types of clients typically recruited for alcoholism treatment studies. Briefly, 80% of the sample was male. The average client was a single, 42-year-old high-school graduate. About half (52%) of the participants were unemployed at the time they were enrolled into the study, and approximately two-thirds (66%) described themselves as single (neither married nor cohabitating with a significant other). Aftercare clients scored significantly higher on measures of alcohol involvement and problem severity than their counterparts in the Outpatient arm. Prior to entering their inpatient treatment programs, participants drank on an average of 22 days per month. On those days when they drank, they typically consumed the equivalent of more than 20 standard drinks (approximately 250 g absolute alcohol), mostly in the form of beer. Sixty-two percent of the sample had been treated previously for alcohol problems, and 98% met *Diagnostic and Statistical Manual*, 3rd edition, revised (DSM-III-R) criteria for alcohol dependence. Clients endorsed an average of 6.8 of the nine DSM-III-R symptoms of alcohol dependence. Many (32%) used illegal substances in addition to alcohol, primarily marijuana. About two-thirds (67%) of participants reported having engaged in alcohol-related criminal behavior, and a sizable minority (40%) admitted to criminal acts unrelated to alcohol use. The average Addiction Severity Index (ASI) Psychiatric Severity score for the sample was 0.23, and 59% had a lifetime Axis I psychiatric disorder. Clearly, this was a sample of severely alcohol-dependent individuals with multiple treatment episodes and some measure of comorbid psychiatric and employment problems. (See Chapter 5 for more detail regarding client characteristics, reasons for exclusion, and sample representativeness.)

Statistical approach

Chapter 7 provides a detailed description of the statistical approach used to test the trial's *a priori* matching hypotheses in both arms of Project MATCH. Briefly, latent growth curve analyses were used to model individual treatment responses (Bryk & Raudenbush, 1987). The active treatment phase (months 1–3) and the post-treatment follow-up period (months 4–15) were analyzed separately. Two primary drinking outcome measures, indices of drinking frequency (Percent Days Abstinent, PDA) and intensity (Drinks per Drinking Day, DDD) were computed for each week of the 12-week treatment phase, and for each month of the 1-year post-treatment follow-up period. Transformations were performed to normalize the distributions of the two drinking indices (arcsin for PDA and square root for DDD). Preliminary model fitting suggested that quadratic curves would adequately account for post-treatment changes in drinking. Separate analyses were conducted for each of the 21 *a priori* matching hypotheses. CRU effects (CRU, CRU by treatment, and CRU by treatment by time) were included as covariate terms in the analytical model, together with the pre-treatment value for each dependent measure (e.g., DDD). A backwards elimination approach was used in the model to test for treatment main effects and for prognostic (main) effects of the matching attributes.

Completion rates for the five follow-up sessions ranged from 93% to 97% and did not differ as a function of treatment assignment. Only 8% of the sample were dropped from the post-treatment analyses due to insufficient data. Additional analyses indicated that the results were not sensitive to missing data exclusion (see Chapter 5 and Project MATCH Research

Group, 1997a, for more information regarding follow-up rates and missing data considerations).

Results

Trends over time

Figures 8.1 and 8.2 show the changes in the two primary outcome measures (PDA and DDD) that occurred over the course of the trial for Aftercare clients in each of the three treatment conditions – Cognitive–Behavioral Therapy (CBT) Motivational Enhancement Therapy (MET), and Twelve Step Facilitation (TSF).

The baseline period refers to a 90-day assessment period prior to entry into the treatment programs from which clients were recruited. As illustrated in Figure 8.1, there was a marked improvement from baseline to the end of treatment for both of the primary drinking outcome measures, and changes in drinking were consistent across the three treatments. The proportion of abstinent days climbed from roughly 25% at baseline to about 90% following treatment (Fig. 8.1), and the number of drinks consumed per occasion was reduced from approximately 20 to about two (Fig. 8.2). This improvement remained relatively consistent and did not decline significantly over the 15-month follow-up period.

Treatment effects

Collapsed across time, there was no significant main effect of treatment on either of the two primary outcome variables during either the active treatment phase or the 1-year post-treatment follow-up period. Within-treatment analyses indicated that a significant treatment by time interaction occurred on the PDA measure. Clients in MET had more abstinent days than those in TSF during weeks 2–4 of treatment, whereas CBT participants reported more abstinent days than those in TSF during weeks 8–11. The time-limited nature of this effect, coupled with the absence of a significant interaction for the DDD variable, suggests that the treatment outcomes for the three therapies were roughly equivalent during the treatment delivery phase. A significant CRU effect was obtained for the PDA outcome measure, indicating that the overall frequency of drinking varied across the five Aftercare sites. However, no significant CRU by treatment

Percent Days Abstinent by Treatment Condition

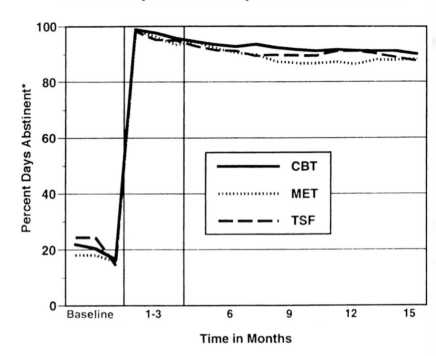

* Estimated from transformed data

Figure 8.1 Monthly Percent Days Abstinent (PDA) for Aftercare clients assigned to Cognitive–Behavioral Therapy (CBT), Motivational Enhancement Therapy (MET) and Twelve Step Facilitation therapy (TSF), for baseline (averaged over 3 months prior to treatment), within treatment (months 1–3), and the year following treatment (months 4–15). (Adapted from Project MATCH Research Group, 1997a.)

effect was found, and no significant site main effects or interaction effects were obtained in analyses of the DDD outcome.

In the post-treatment follow-up period, a small but statistically significant treatment by linear time effect emerged in an analysis that included adjustments for the 10 primary matching hypothesis attributes: TSF clients reported fewer drinking days (PDA) toward the end of the follow-up period. However, no treatment differences were observed in the analysis of the drinking intensity measure (DDD). Given the presence of CRU by treatment interactions and the results of the primary (unadjusted)

Drinks per Drinking Day by Treatment Condition

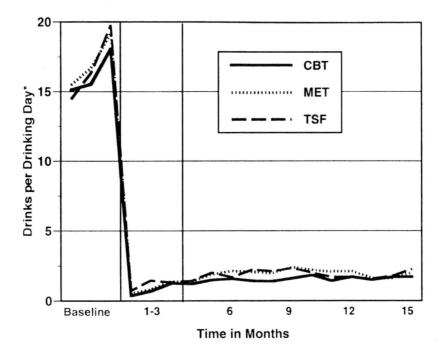

* **Estimated from transformed data**

Figure 8.2 Monthly Drinks per Drinking Day (DDD) for Aftercare clients assigned to Cognitive–Behavioral Therapy (CBT), Motivational Enhancement Therapy (MET) and Twelve Step Facilitation therapy (TSF), at baseline (averaged over 3 months prior to treatment), within treatment (months 1–3), and the year following treatment (months 4–15). (Adapted from Project MATCH Research Group, 1997a.)

analyses, it was concluded that there were no clinically significant differences in primary drinking outcomes among the three treatments (see Chapter 7 and Project MATCH Research Group, 1997a, regarding site effects). Thus, the demonstrated improvements from baseline drinking levels shown in Figure 8.1 were generally quite consistent across treatment modalities during both the active treatment phase and the post-treatment follow-up period.

Table 8.1. *Significant post-treatment prognostic effects of primary and*
secondary matching attributes on primary drinking outcomes[a]

	Percent Days Abstinent	Drinks per Drinking Day
Primary matching variable		
Alcohol Involvement		+
Gender (male versus female)	−	+
Support for Drinking		+
Secondary matching variable		
Religiosity	+	
Self-efficacy		
Temptation minus Confidence	−	+

[a]Only main (non-time-dependent) effects are shown. Entries indicate the direction of the prognostic main effect, with a blank space indicating no significant effect in that category. Additional details regarding the nature of these effects can be found in primary sources (Project MATCH Research Group, 1997a; 1997b).

Prognostic effects

In addition to treatment effects, it is important to know whether the matching attributes selected for study had any prognostic effects of their own that might allow a prediction of treatment outcome. The results of the analyses examining main effects (not dependent on time) for the primary and secondary matching variables in the Aftercare arm are summarized in Table 8.1. Of the ten primary matching characteristics, only Gender predicted both PDA and DDD over the entire 1-year follow-up period. As might be expected, male clients had more drinking days, and consumed more alcohol on those days, than their female counterparts. In addition, more serious Alcohol Involvement and more Support for Drinking were associated with higher consumption on drinking occasions.

Only two of the secondary hypothesis matching attributes, Religiosity and one of the two Self-efficacy measures (Temptation minus Confidence) produced significant prognostic effects, and only the latter variable demonstrated a consistent effect on both primary drinking outcome variables. Stronger Religiosity was associated with less frequent drinking (PDA). Clients who reported higher levels of temptation to drink prior to treatment, coupled with lower levels of perceived efficacy to abstain, had poorer PDA and DDD outcomes (Project MATCH Research Group, 1997b).

Tests of matching hypotheses

The results of the tests of the 21 *a priori* hypotheses for the Aftercare study are summarized in Table 8.2. As shown in the table, none of the primary *a priori* matching contrasts was significant (i.e., yielding a statistically significant attribute by treatment interaction, ATI) in the predicted direction using the Bonferroni-corrected *alpha* level during either the phase of active treatment or the post-treatment follow-up period. However, significant ATI by linear time effects were obtained for Meaning Seeking for PDA (but not DDD) and for Typology for DDD (but not PDA) in analyses of the 1-year follow-up period. More specifically, during the latter half of the follow-up period, clients in the TSF condition who had higher baseline Meaning Seeking scores reported proportionately more abstinent days than clients in either the CBT or MET treatment groups. With regard to Typology, no single monthly contrast reached the 0.05 level of significance, although the three-way interaction (attribute by treatment by time) was significant (see Project MATCH Research Group, 1997a).

As shown in Table 8.2, two of the secondary hypothesis matching variables, both measures of Self-efficacy (Confidence, and Temptation minus Confidence), produced significant matching effects during the treatment phase. Whereas the Confidence measure resulted in a significant ATI for both PDA and DDD, the Temptation minus Confidence measure only reached statistical significance for the DDD outcome, and the effect was time dependent. Neither Self-efficacy variable produced significant matching effects in the analyses of the post-treatment period.

A significant ATI was obtained for both of the primary drinking outcome measures in the post-treatment analyses for the matching hypothesis variable Alcohol Dependence. CBT clients who reported lower levels of dependence drank less frequently and consumed smaller quantities than those in the TSF condition. The reverse occurred for participants with more severe dependence on alcohol: among these clients, those treated in the TSF condition drank less often and had fewer drinks per occasion than those in CBT (Fig. 8.3). Thus, highly dependent clients benefited more from TSF, whereas their less dependent counterparts fared better in CBT.

A positive matching effect was also observed for participants with an Antisocial Personality Disorder (ASPD) diagnosis, but only for one drinking outcome measure (DDD), and this time-dependent effect was not consistent over the entire post-treatment period. In addition, significant matching effects (not listed in the table) were found for the secondary

Table 8.2. *Statistically significant treatment matching effects across time*

Matching hypothesis	Treatment contrast	Drinking outcome	Within-treatment effect	Post-treatment effect
Primary matching variable				
Meaning seeking	TSF vs. (CBT & MET)	PDA		ATI[a] × time
Typology	MET vs. CBT	DDD		ATI × time
Secondary matching variable				
Alcohol dependence	CBT vs. TSF	PDA		ATI
		DDD		ATI
Antisocial Personality Disorder	CBT vs. MET	DDD		ATI × time
	CBT vs. TSF	DDD		ATI × time
Self-efficacy				
Confidence	MET vs. CBT	PDA	ATI	
		DDD	ATI	
	MET vs. TSF	PDA	ATI	
		DDD	ATI	
Temptation minus Confidence	MET vs. TSF	DDD	ATI × time	

[a] ATI = Attribute by Treatment Interaction. See text for details regarding methods of analysis. Additional details regarding the nature of the effects listed in this table can be found in primary sources (Project MATCH Research Group, 1997a; 1997b; 1998b).

TSF, Twelve Step Facilitation; CBT, Cognitive–Behavioral Therapy; MET, Motivational Enhancement Therapy; PDA, Percent Days Abstinent; DDD, Drinks per Drinking Day.

Alcohol Dependence Matching Effect

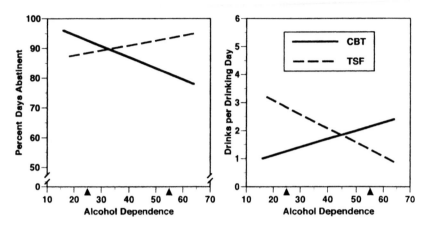

Figure 8.3 Alcohol Dependence matching effect during the year following treatment (months 4–15). Cognitive–Behavioral Therapy (CBT) contrasted with Twelve Step Facilitation therapy (TSF) on two primary outcome measures, Percent of Days Abstinent (PDA) and Drinks per Drinking Day (DDD). (Copyright 1997, Society for the Study of Addiction to Alcohol and Other Drugs. Adapted with permission from Project MATCH Research Group, 1997b, p. 1683.)

matching characteristics, Prior Engagement in Alcoholics Anonymous and Readiness to Change, in the direction opposite to that specified by the hypotheses. Previous AA involvement, coupled with assignment to TSF, resulted in more drinks per drinking day during the final 3 weeks of treatment. For the Readiness to Change hypothesis, MET, as compared with CBT, was associated with more drinking during treatment for clients lower in readiness, but the effect diminished over time in the follow-up period (Project MATCH Research Group, 1997b).

Exploratory analyses

The exploratory analysis strategies described in Chapter 7 using the 20 predictor variable set and 15 Alcohol Use Inventory (AUI) subscale scores (see Table 7.3) were repeated for the Aftercare sample. In these analyses, an additional measure, Length of Stay (total number of days in inpatient/ day-hospital treatment prior to aftercare), was included. No significant interactions were found when the variables were entered into hierarchical regression analyses of the two primary drinking outcome measures. Thus, exploratory analyses using the Aftercare sample found little evidence for additional matches between client variables and treatment condition. As in the Outpatient study, the possibility of other matching effects cannot be ruled out. However, any large, significant matching effects should have emerged in these analyses.

Causal chain analyses and clinical significance of matching

Only one of the *a priori* matching hypotheses, Alcohol Dependence, produced an unqualified effect (i.e., not time dependent) during the year-long post-treatment follow-up period. Consistent with the hypothesis, severely dependent clients benefited more from TSF than from CBT, while the reverse was true for less alcohol-dependent participants. (A parallel hypothesis involving a TSF versus MET contrast was not supported.) The causal chain for this hypothesis specified two possible mechanisms underlying the effect.

First, it was anticipated that TSF therapists would emphasize abstinence as a treatment goal more than CBT therapists, who would instead provide more explicit instructions regarding coping with lapses. Highly dependent participants were expected to do poorly in CBT because their coping skills would be inadequate for dealing with lapses. Given their high levels of dependence and previous experiences with drinking, re-initiation of alcohol use was expected to result in a rapid re-instatement of symptoms. On the other hand, it was predicted that less dependent clients would use the lapse-coping skills acquired in CBT more effectively, while reacting negatively to the AA notion of loss of control, which was likely to be inconsistent with their own drinking histories. Analyses of treatment process data for the Aftercare arm supported the prediction that TSF therapists emphasized abstinence more as a treatment goal. Further, less dependent clients reported higher proportions of abstinent days when assigned to therapists who did not emphasize abstinence, whereas more severely dependent participants had similar outcomes regardless of the degree of emphasis on abstinence (Cooney et al., 2001).

Second, the Alcohol Dependence hypothesis predicted a mediating role for AA attendance and involvement. More severely dependent clients were expected to attend more AA sessions and to become more involved in AA activities than those who were less alcohol dependent, and AA participation was anticipated to be more strongly associated with lower rates of drinking in the more dependent clients. Only partial support was found for this set of predictions. Dependence severity was a strong predictor of AA attendance, which, in turn, was strongly related to drinking outcomes. However, there was no evidence for an Alcohol Dependence by AA attendance interaction effect. That is, the posited causal chain did not explain the Alcohol Dependence matching effect.

To evaluate the clinical significance of the Alcohol Dependence matching effect, clients were assigned to 'success' and 'failure' outcome categories for each follow-up evaluation, and a cut-off score was used to further partition clients into two groups (high and low) based on their Alcohol Dependence scores. As described more fully in the preceding chapter, a successful treatment outcome was defined as abstinence or moderate drinking without alcohol-related problems during the 3-month follow-up intervals; outcome was classified as a failure when a participant reported any heavy drinking and/or negative consequences. Highly dependent clients were considered to be appropriately matched if randomly assigned to TSF and mismatched if assigned to CBT; conversely, clients in the low dependence group were seen as matched in CBT and mismatched in TSF. The results of this analysis showed that the maximum matching effect occurred 6–12 months after the initiation of treatment. Matched clients had roughly a 10% higher success rate than mismatched clients, and a 5% higher success rate than unmatched or randomly assigned clients.

Discussion

Overall, Aftercare clients improved significantly from baseline through the 15-month follow-up period, both in the frequency and in the intensity of drinking, and these improvements did not vary as a function of treatment condition. More germane to the purpose of Project MATCH, there was evidence for only one robust matching effect. Participants who were highly dependent on alcohol had better post-treatment outcomes in TSF, whereas less severely dependent clients fared better in CBT.

The reasons why more of the matching effects observed in previous single-site studies with smaller sample sizes (see Mattson et al., 1994, for a review) were not found in the present research are unclear. Given the large sample size ($n = 774$, with more than 200 clients in each of the three treatment conditions) and the number of matching effects tested (31 planned treatment contrasts for 21 *a priori* matching variables), it is surprising that more statistically significant effects did not occur by chance. Marked CRU main effects were observed in both arms of the trial for both the active treatment phase (Project MATCH Research Group, 1998b) and the 1-year follow-up period (Project MATCH Research Group, 1997a), suggesting that conclusions from single-site studies might be misleading. However, site-by-site tests of matching hypotheses indicated that the negative matching results were generalizable across CRUs.

One possible reason for the relative lack of matching effects is that the wrong matching attributes were chosen for evaluation. This is unlikely, given the large number of *a priori* matching hypotheses that were evaluated and the fact that many of the matching variables (e.g., Typology, Psychiatric Severity, Conceptual Level) were based upon previous reports in the literature (McLachlan, 1972; McLellan et al., 1983; Litt et al., 1992). Moreover, exploratory analyses using 36 additional predictor variables found little evidence of matches between client variables and treatment condition that might have been missed by focusing on only the *a priori* matching attributes.

Fewer significant matching effects were obtained in the Aftercare arm of the trial than in the Outpatient study (Project MATCH Research Group, 1997a; 1997b; 1998a, 1998b). Several factors may have accounted for this difference. Aftercare participants were recruited from a population of clients who had completed a formal inpatient or day-hospital treatment program. Factors associated with this experience may have masked potential matching effects. For example, the treatment programs imposed a period of sobriety ranging from 7 to 44 days immediately prior to entry into Project MATCH; perhaps only the most highly motivated clients were able to meet this requirement for completion of the inpatient programs.

Another difference between the two arms of the trial concerns the nature of the prior treatment that Aftercare clients received as inpatients. As noted above, AA philosophy and attendance were major components of most of the inpatient treatment programs. Thus, even before entering Project MATCH, the Aftercare participants had been instructed about the need to remain sober, and many had also received some type of relapse prevention therapy. For the Aftercare sample, *maintaining* abstinence was the aim of treatment, whereas for Outpatient clients, *attaining* sobriety was the goal. These factors may explain why Aftercare participants were much more likely to attend AA meetings than their Outpatient counterparts throughout the trial, regardless of their Project MATCH group assignment (see Chapter 11). It is possible that the high degree of therapeutic intervention and AA inculcation among Aftercare clients prior to participation in the trial may have masked any treatment matching effects. The one significant matching effect in the Aftercare arm for the Alcohol Dependence hypothesis underscores the important role that AA principles may play in the maintenance of sobriety, particularly for severely dependent clients.

Recently, it has been suggested that a history of *previous* AA attendance is not necessarily related to more successful treatment outcome or prognosis (Humphreys et al., 1998). A more important variable may be the difference in AA attendance *during* treatment. As compared to the Aftercare arm, AA attendance in the Outpatient sample varied much more markedly as a function of treatment assignment, which may have allowed for the emergence of differential main effects and matching results. When there was a treatment effect in the Outpatient arm, it was always in favor of TSF (Project MATCH Research Group, 1997a, 1998b).

Finally, it is possible that the positive outcomes observed throughout the course of the trial created a ceiling effect that reduced the likelihood that treatment or matching effects would emerge. The fact that an inpatient treatment episode followed by intensive aftercare for 12 weeks and regular follow-up evaluations was so successful in maintaining favorable outcomes should be considered a significant finding in its own right. It is not possible to determine whether the positive outcomes were sustained by the Aftercare treatments *per se*, by the follow-up evaluations conducted every 3 months by a concerned research assistant, or by a combination of the two. Nevertheless, 35% of the Aftercare clients remained totally abstinent during the 1-year follow-up period, which is a clinically significant finding.

9

Treatment effects across multiple dimensions of outcome

THOMAS F. BABOR, KAREN STEINBERG, ALLEN ZWEBEN,
RON CISLER, ROBERT STOUT, J. SCOTT TONIGAN,
RAYMOND F. ANTON, AND JOHN P. ALLEN

Changes in the quantity (Percent Days Abstinent, PDA) and intensity (Drinks per Drinking Day, DDD) of drinking reported in Chapters 7 and 8 raise important questions about the extent to which the Project MATCH treatments were associated with changes in alternative measures of drinking as well as improvements in other areas of life such as psychological, physical, and social functioning. To provide a more comprehensive view of treatment outcomes, this chapter begins with an evaluation of the effects of treatment on three alternative types of drinking outcomes: time to first drinking event, a composite outcome measure that encompasses alcohol problems as well as the amount of drinking, and a combined 'clean and sober' measure that reflects both drug and alcohol use. Another set of analyses examines the effects of the three treatments on measures of other drug use: liver function, alcohol-related consequences, social role performance, psychopathology, depression, and days working. The findings indicate significant improvements in outcome status from baseline to follow-up on all measures. With one notable exception, the improvements following treatment were not related to treatment condition or study arm. On measures relating to continuous abstinence, there was a consistent treatment effect favoring Twelve Step Facilitation in both arms of the trial. Finally, the results show that the lower the level of post-treatment alcohol consumption, the greater the improvement observed in other areas of life functioning.

Although drinking is the *sine qua non* of alcohol-related problems, a narrow focus on the frequency and intensity of drinking leaves many questions unanswered about the effects of treatment on physical health and psychosocial well-being. Does Cognitive–Behavioral Therapy (CBT) relieve depression and other general psychiatric impairment better than other treatments? Does the Twelve Step Faciliation (TSF), with its emphasis on total abstinence, lead to superior outcomes in physical health, such as improved liver function? Does the Motivational Enhancement Therapy (MET) encourage alcoholics to reduce their use of other drugs in addition to alcohol? The purpose of this chapter is to describe the changes observed in Project MATCH clients in a variety of life areas during and after treatment, and to consider how treatment affected drinking patterns measured in ways other than quantity and frequency of alcohol use. In addition, this chapter describes how changes and reductions in drinking behavior during the follow-up period may be related to improvements in important areas of life functioning such as mood, work, health, other drug use, and social functioning.

There has been some contention about whether the effects of alcoholism treatment should be evaluated solely against the criterion of complete abstinence (Pattison et al., 1977). On the one hand, the unitary view of alcoholism argues that total abstinence from alcohol is the best indicator of successful response to treatment, based on the assumption that improvement in psychosocial functioning and physical health necessarily depends on sobriety (Babor et al., 1989). On the other hand, it could be argued that abstinence may not affect all measures of outcome status, such as employment or marital relationships, because these dimensions are independent of drinking behavior, particularly in people with poor occupational or interpersonal skills (McLellan et al., 1981). Consistent with this view is the tendency to assess a broad range of life areas in treatment evaluation research, such as physical health, other substance use, legal problems, vocational functioning, social adjustment, and psychological status.

Treatment evaluation studies provide limited support for both the unitary and multidimensional views. For example, Babor et al. (1989) evaluated 266 treated alcoholics on a variety of outcome dimensions over a 3-year period. Although different outcome dimensions were only moderately correlated with each other, there was a clear linear relationship between post-treatment drinking and lack of improvement in medical status, biological function, life stress, and psychopathology. To date, the evidence does not uniformly support either the unitary or the multidimensional approach to the characterization of treatment outcome, nor does it provide more than suggestive evidence linking changes in drinking directly to improvements in other areas of functioning during the course of recovery following treatment.

To provide a more comprehensive view of treatment outcomes in Project MATCH, this chapter begins with an evaluation of two types of alternative drinking outcomes: time to first drinking event and a composite outcome measure. It was expected that these measures would provide valuable information about the effects of the three treatments on the duration of abstinence, patterns of relapse, and the problems experienced in relation to drinking. A third measure was developed to assess whether the three treatments differentially affected the extent to which clients were 'clean and sober' at follow-up, i.e., abstinent from illict drugs as well as alcohol.

Another set of analyses examines the effects of the three treatments on selected outcome variables considered to be important secondary benefits of treatment. These alternative outcome measures provide a more complete picture of the effects of treatment than the primary drinking measures alone (described in Chapters 7 and 8). The measures include the liver function test, gamma-glutamyl transpeptidase (GGTP), as well as assessments of drinking-related consequences, work involvement, depression, psychiatric severity, and illicit drug use. The chapter concludes with an analysis of the relation between drinking and psychosocial functioning during the follow-up period, which speaks to the critical issue of whether the reduction or cessation of drinking following treatment is associated with improvements in a variety of different life areas.

Methods

Measures of life functioning and psychological status were included in the assessment battery to study the effects of treatment matching on the lives of the study participants (see Chapter 3). These secondary measures of physical health, social role functioning, and psychological status were assessed both at baseline and at the 3-month, 9-month, 15-month, and 39-month (for Outpatient participants) follow-up points.

The primary interview used to measure drinking behavior, the Form-90, contained a variety of ways to define drinking outcomes, other than the frequency (Percent Days Abstinent, PDA) and intensity (Drinks per Drinking Day, DDD) of alcohol use. These alternative ways to assess drinking following treatment included three duration measures: (1) time to first drink, defined as the consumption of any amount of alcohol; (2) time to first day of 'heavy' drinking; and (3) time to first day when three successive 'heavy' drinking days in a row were observed. The definition of heavy drinking was gender specific: consumption of six or more standard drinks over 24 hours for males, and of four or more standard drinks for women. The first-drink criterion reflects a traditional, strict standard for treatment success or failure. Consumption of a single drink, however, does not necessarily suggest a catastrophic outcome in the near future; the heavy-drinking criterion reflects a level of consumption at which concern about future outcome would be considerably higher. A single day of drinking at the heavy level, however, might still be considered under some circumstances to be more of a 'lapse' than a 'relapse.' Thus, the third criterion, three successive days of heavy drinking, was added to represent a level of drinking that almost all clinicians would regard as a clear relapse.

In addition to terminal drinking events, a Composite outcome measure was developed (Zweben & Cisler, 1996; Cisler & Zweben, 1999), based on the recognition that independent measures of alcohol use and related problems do not capture the full complexity of relapse following participation in treatment (Duckitt et al., 1985). Evidence has shown that alcoholics may have differing levels of alcohol problem severity despite having similar consumption patterns (Zweben & Cisler, 1996). Some individuals may have the social, psychological, and economic resources to mitigate against the negative effects of drinking, whereas others have few coping resources.

Using conceptually derived cut-off criteria for alcohol use and related consequences as measured by the Drinker Inventory of Consequences (DrInC; Miller et al., 1995b), summary scores were used to assign individuals to four composite categories at intake, and again at each of the follow-up points. The four levels for this variable were: (1) no drinking; (2) moderate drinking and nonrecurrent problems; (3) heavy drinking or recurrent problems; and (4) both heavy drinking and recurrent problems. The composite measure takes into account events occurring during the most recent 3 months, and combines alcohol consumption and alcohol-related problems into a single, graduated treatment outcome classification.

The DrInC was also employed in other analyses as a continuous measure of the totality of alcohol-related intrapersonal, interpersonal, and physical consequences. The Addiction Severity Index (ASI: McLellan et al., 1992) was used to measure changes in psychiatric severity, and the Beck Depression Inventory (Beck et al., 1986) was administered to measure the severity of depressive symptomatology. The Form-90 (Miller, 1996) provided a measure of days working and use of drugs other than alcohol over the previous 90 days. GGTP was used to measure the effects of alcohol on liver function. The Psychosocial Functioning Inventory (PFI: Feragne et al., 1983) measured the client's competence in meeting important social role demands.

Results

Alternative measures of drinking behavior

Figure 9.1 shows 'survival curves,' which represent the proportion of clients who avoided 'relapse' as a function of time from the nominal end of treatment, which is day 90 in the study, a time when most participants would have completed the treatment phase. Therefore, the time axis of Figure 9.1 represents the number of days after day 90. As the two panels show, relapse rates are highest in both arms immediately after treatment (some clients were actually drinking at the end of treatment and were counted as having relapsed immediately), as indicated by the steep drop in the survival curves. As time progresses, the rate of new relapses decreases and the curves tend to flatten. The estimated number of relapses increases as the criterion for relapse becomes more stringent. The proportion of failures in the Outpatient arm is uniformly higher than in the Aftercare arm. However, this difference tends to decrease as the criterion for failure is made less stringent. The survival rates after 1 year at risk are indicated on the figure. In the Outpatient arm, about 16% of subjects avoided taking a drink in the year after treatment, while in the Aftercare arm 30% avoided doing so. For three successive drinking days, however, the difference narrows to 48% versus 55%, respectively.

Using proportional hazards analyses (Cox, 1972), significant effects were found among the Outpatient clients for time to first drink ($p < 0.001$). TSF clients had the best outcome on this measure, with 24% avoiding any drinking in months 4–15, whereas the corresponding figures for CBT and MET were 15% and 14%, respectively. When we analyzed the more stringent criteria of first heavy drinking and three successive days of heavy drinking, treatment main effects were also significant. Once again, the TSF condition had the better outcomes, with 53% not reaching the three heavy drinking days criterion, followed by MET with 49% and CBT with 48%. There were no statistically significant treatment main effects in the outcomes of the Aftercare clients.

Figure 9.2 shows how Aftercare and Outpatient clients were classified according to the four composite outcome categories. In the Outpatient group, almost all of the clients were classified as heavy drinkers with recurrent problems during the 3 months prior to treatment. Following treatment, the proportion of heavy drinkers with problems diminished considerably, to roughly 40% at each of the follow-up time points. Proportions of Outpatients in the other three drinking categories remained fairly

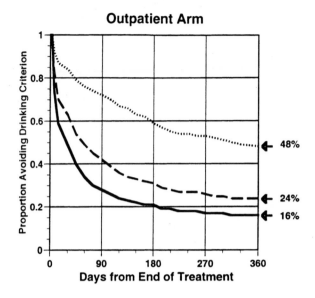

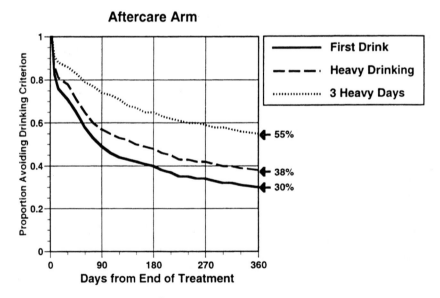

Figure 9.1 Time to three types of relapse events (first drink, first heavy drinking, first episode of three heavy drinking days) for Outpatient arm and Aftercare arm.

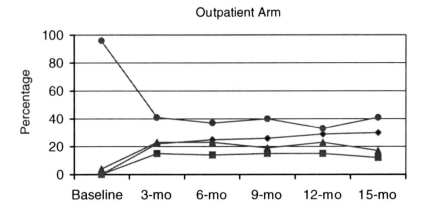

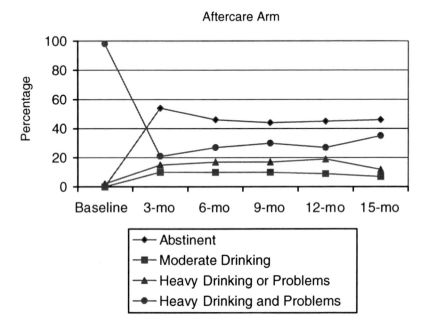

Figure 9.2 Percentages of Outpatient and Aftercare clients classified according to four composite outcome categories at baseline and at five follow-up points.

consistent after treatment ended, with between 20% and 30% (depending on the follow-up time point) remaining abstinent.

As with the Outpatients, virtually all of the Aftercare clients were classified as 'heavy drinking with recurrent problems' at baseline and showed dramatic improvements after treatment (Fig. 9.2). However, the Aftercare group had a greater percentage of 'abstinent' participants, averaging over 40% at each follow-up period, and a corresponding lower proportion of clients in the most severe category.

This dramatic change among both groups from baseline to the 3-month interview suggests that entry into treatment or treatment itself had an immediate impact. Moreover, the proportion of clients in different categories remained relatively consistent throughout the 1-year follow-up (although individual clients showed considerable variation in classification), with Aftercare clients showing greater levels of abstinence and lower proportions of heavy drinking with problems.

In log-linear analyses of the composite measure (Project MATCH Research Group, 1997a), treatment main effects were significant at month 15 ($p < 0.01$) for Outpatient clients. The difference was due to a higher percentage of TSF clients in the abstinent category, relative to the percentages for the CBT and MET clients. There were no treatment differences in the Aftercare arm.

Similar treatment main effects were obtained when alcohol and illicit drug use were jointly considered in a single measure reflecting client substance use. At each follow-up period, clients were assigned to one of four categories: (1) completely abstinent from alcohol *and* illicit drugs; (2) use of illicit drugs but no alcohol consumption; (3) use of alcohol but no illicit drugs; and (4) use of *both* alcohol and illicit drugs. Logistic regressions were conducted to evaluate this 'clean and sober' variable (group 1 versus groups 2, 3, and 4) separately for Aftercare and Outpatient samples. Controlling for site variation and baseline alcohol and drug use, the treatment main effect probabilities for the five follow-up periods in the Outpatient arm were: $p < 0.07$, $p < 0.004$, $p < 0.026$, $p < 0.028$, and $p < 0.176$. TSF clients reported significantly higher rates of complete abstinence from substances relative to MET and CBT clients at the 6-month, 9-month, and 12-month follow-up points. Parallel statistical analyses indicated no treatment main effect on multiple substance use at any of the five follow-up points in the Aftercare arm.

Secondary outcome measures

Analyses of secondary outcome measures involved two 3-month time periods: months 7–9 and 13–15 (Project MATCH Research Group, 1997a). These periods were chosen because many of the outcome measures were assessed during the in-person interviews conducted at months 9 and 15. Continuous outcome variables were analyzed by repeated measures analysis of covariance. In these analyses, the baseline value of the dependent measure was used as a covariate. The analyses also adjusted for site effects and for the interaction between site and treatment condition.

The outcomes evaluated in this analysis were Days Working, Psychiatric Severity, Alcohol-related Consequences, GGTP, Depression, Social Functioning, and Drug Use. For the Drug Use variable, logistic regression was used. Because most illegal substances, other than marijuana, were used infrequently, a binary outcome measure, 'use of any illegal substance,' was created.

The analyses indicated significant improvements in outcome status from baseline to follow-up on all measures in both arms of the trial. Almost all of the gains were evident at the end of treatment, with little change thereafter. These results are illustrated in Figure 9.3 for the Outpatient and Aftercare clients. In comparison to Aftercare clients, Outpatients reported more Days Working, less Psychiatric Severity, less Depression, and a greater amount of other Drug Use (most often marijuana) at baseline and throughout the 12-month follow-up period.

With one exception, the universal improvements following treatment were not related to treatment condition or study arm. TSF clients in the Outpatient arm had significantly fewer drinking consequences than clients in the other two treatments at month 9, but at month 15 the three treatments did not differ significantly (Project MATCH Research Group, 1997a).

Inter-relatedness of secondary outcome measures

We assessed the degree to which the secondary outcome dimensions constituting relatively independent domains demonstrated statistical independence. Correlational analyses at baseline and 15-month follow-up generally confirmed the relative independence of these secondary outcome dimensions. Although many of the correlations were statistically significant, the magnitude of the associations was in the low to moderate range

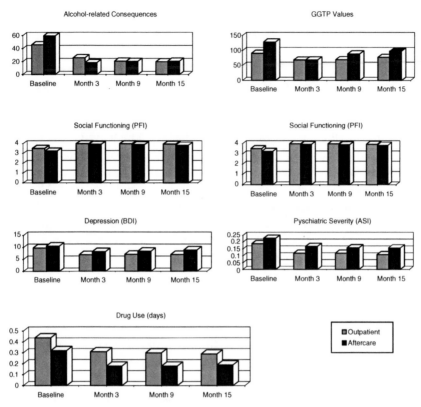

Figure 9.3 Secondary outcome measures at baseline and follow-up for Outpatient and Aftercare participants.

(i.e., 0.10–0.30) for most variables. Secondary outcome dimensions with the strongest associations (in the range of 0.40–0.70) were those that were conceptually similar (e.g., Depression and Psychiatric Severity).

Relation between post-treatment drinking and secondary outcome measures

Although there were virtually no differences among the three treatment groups in the post-treatment measures of secondary outcomes, there were large improvements across all conditions on these measures from baseline to follow-up. That is, both drinking and secondary outcome variables changed over time, and these changes seemed to correspond to one another. These findings are consistent with the hypothesis that improvements across these domains were, in part, related to the reductions in drinking from baseline to follow-up. In order to further explore this hypothesis, we first examined the cross-sectional relationships between drinking and secondary outcomes.

Table 9.1 shows the correlations between primary drinking measures (PDA and DDD) and secondary outcomes at baseline and 15-month follow-up. In general, the table shows that: (1) correlations were stronger at follow-up than during baseline assessment; (2) DDD was more closely related to the secondary outcomes than PDA; and (3) correlations were stronger for Aftercare clients and females than for Outpatients and males. The secondary outcomes most strongly related to drinking were Alcohol-related Consequences, Depression, and Social Role Performance. These findings suggest that the secondary outcomes are related to drinking levels during the post-treatment period. However, secondary outcomes are differentially associated with the frequency and intensity of drinking.

These cross-sectional relationships beg the question: to what extent are these measures of physical and psychosocial functioning assessed at the 15-month follow-up point related to changes in drinking that had taken place earlier? Multiple regression analyses were conducted to examine the prospective contribution of post-treatment drinking to secondary outcome dimensions (Alcohol-related Consequences, Drug Use, GGTP, Social Functioning, Depression, Psychiatric Severity, and Days Working) at the 15-month follow-up. These analyses controlled for the effects of demographics (age, gender, ethnicity, marital status, and level of education), baseline drinking, treatment condition (MET, TSF, CBT), and interim functioning (9-month follow-up). Linear regressions were performed hierarchically, entering variables in the following order: (1) demographics, (2) baseline drinking levels, (3) baseline functioning (for the particular secondary outcome measure being regressed), (4) treatment condition, (5) interim functioning (for regressed secondary outcome variable), and (6) drinking at previous assessment. This approach evaluates the unique contribution of post-treatment drinking in the 3 months prior to the 15-month follow-up, after controlling for the influence of demographic factors, prior drinking, prior functioning, treatment received, and post-treatment interim functioning. Table 9.2 shows the changes in total variance accounted for at each step for each of the secondary outcome measures. The results show that Alcohol-related Consequences, Depression, Social Functioning, and Drug Use are significantly related to alcohol consumption after controlling for a variety of other possible influences. Although the increment in

Table 9.1. *Cross-sectional correlations between primary measures of drinking – Percent Days Abstinent (PDA), Drinks per Drinking Day (DDD) – and seven secondary outcome measures according to study arm and gender*

		Outpatient				Aftercare			
		Male		Female		Male		Female	
		PDA	DDD	PDA	DDD	PDA	DDD	PDA	DDD
Alcohol-related consequences	Baseline	-0.14[b]	0.38[b]	-0.07	0.29[b]	-0.09[a]	0.34[b]	0.01	0.50[b]
	15 months	-0.48[b]	0.63[b]	-0.50[b]	0.68[b]	-0.53[b]	0.64[b]	-0.54[b]	0.70[b]
GGTP	Baseline	-0.18[b]	0.07	-0.19	0.11	-0.20[b]	0.08	-0.17[a]	0.21[b]
	15 months	-0.17[b]	0.23[b]	-0.21[b]	0.16[a]	-0.34[b]	0.27[b]	-0.30[b]	0.35[b]
Days Working	Baseline	0.01	-0.03[b]	0.02	-0.19[b]	-0.03	-0.16[b]	-0.13	-0.17[a]
	15 months	-0.07	-0.07	-0.02	-0.12	0.02	-0.16[b]	0.12	-0.21[a]
Depression	Baseline	-0.10[b]	0.13[b]	0.01	0.23[b]	0.02	0.22[b]	0.05	0.28[b]
	15 months	-0.23[b]	0.32[b]	-0.27[b]	0.38[b]	-0.28[b]	0.37[b]	-0.32[b]	0.39[b]
Psychiatric Severity	Baseline	-0.03	0.15[b]	-0.02	0.08	0.04	0.07	0.09	0.20[a]
	15 months	0.01	0.13[b]	-0.10	0.20[b]	-0.15[b]	0.28[b]	-0.27	0.29[b]
Drug use	Baseline	0.01	0.06	-0.01	0.11	-0.02	0.05	0.01	0.06
	15 months	-0.12[b]	0.20[b]	-0.10	0.18[b]	-0.20[b]	0.24[b]	-0.33[b]	0.22[b]
Social Functioning	Baseline	0.05	-0.14[b]	0.10	-0.16[b]	-0.04	-0.09[a]	0.05	-0.16
	15 months	0.19[b]	-0.32	0.25[b]	-0.34[b]	0.23[b]	-0.28[b]	0.20[a]	-0.33[b]

[a] $p < 0.05$.
[b] $p < 0.01$.
GGTP, serum gamma-glutamyl transpeptidase.

Table 9.2. *Hierarchical multivariate linear regression results for secondary outcome measures in Outpatient arm and Aftercare arm*

Step[a]	Depression	Social functioning	Psychiatric severity	Alcohol-related consequences	GGTP	Drug use	Days working
Outpatient							
1	0.02[b]	0.00	0.03[c]	0.01	0.04[d]	0.11[d]	0.11[d]
2	0.04[c]	0.01	0.03	0.03[c]	0.04	0.11	0.13[d]
3	0.27[d]	0.10[d]	0.10[d]	0.05[c]	0.39[d]	0.25[d]	0.32[d]
4	0.27	0.10	0.10	0.06[e]	0.39	0.25	0.32
5	0.43[d]	0.31[d]	0.32[d]	0.40[d]	0.55[d]	0.46[d]	0.41[d]
6	0.44[d]	0.32[d]	0.32	0.45[d]	0.56[e]	0.47[e]	0.41[b]
Aftercare							
1	0.01	0.03[c]	0.02[b]	0.04[c]	0.03[c]	0.08[d]	0.13[d]
2	0.02[b]	0.03	0.02	0.04	0.04[b]	0.08	0.14[e]
3	0.15[d]	0.06[d]	0.10[d]	0.07[d]	0.25[d]	0.18[d]	0.23[d]
4	0.15	0.07	0.10	0.07	0.26	0.18	0.24
5	0.36[d]	0.25[d]	0.30[d]	0.30[d]	0.57[d]	0.32[d]	0.37[d]
6	0.39[d]	0.27[c]	0.30	0.40[d]	0.58	0.34[d]	0.38

[a] Step 1: demographics (age, gender, ethnicity, education, marital status).
Step 2: baseline drinking (PDA, DDD).
Step 3: baseline value of secondary outcome measure.
Step 4: treatment condition (CBT, MET, TSF).
Step 5: interim value of secondary outcome measure.
Step 6: interim values of drinking measures (PDA, DDD).
Note: Cumulative R^2 for each step is reported.
[b] $= p < 0.05$.
[c] $p < 0.01$.
[d] $p < 0.001$.
[e] $p < 0.1$.
GGTP, Serum gamma-glutamyl transpeptidase; PDA, Percent Days Abstinent; DDD, Drinks per Drinking Day; CBT, Cognitive–Behavioral Therapy; MET, Motivational Enhancement Therapy; TSF, Twelve Step Facilitation.

variance accounted for by alcohol consumption is in the modest range (R^2 changes ranged from 0.01 to 0.10), it is noteworthy that post-treatment drinking was predictive of later functioning.

Discussion

This chapter examines two major issues related to alcoholism treatment outcome. First, how did the Project MATCH treatments affect alternative measures of drinking behavior (i.e., survival measures and a composite outcome) and seven secondary outcome dimensions that cover different aspects of life functioning? Second, how are changes in drinking related to improvements in post-treatment functioning in a variety of life areas related to health and social adjustment?

Effects of treatment

There were several significant treatment main effects on alternative measures of drinking behavior in the Outpatient arm for time to first drinking events and the composite outcome. TSF was shown to be superior to both CBT and MET. In addition, Outpatient TSF clients evidenced much higher rates of continuous abstinence during the follow-up period (24% as compared with 15% for CBT and 14% for MET clients). Although all three interventions encouraged abstinence as a goal of treatment, it may be that the abstinence philosophy and social support aspects underlying the AA-based TSF approach produce greater abstinence, and this seems to be associated with improvements in other areas of functioning. We have seen throughout Project MATCH other factors related to TSF that may be important in designing future interventions and tailoring treatments for particular clients. For example, clients who showed less psychiatric severity appeared to benefit more from TSF than from CBT (Project MATCH Research Group, 1997a). TSF clients were more likely to be involved in AA, and those who benefited most from TSF were individuals who had social networks that were supportive of their drinking prior to treatment (Longabaugh et al., 1998). Thus, the benefits associated with TSF appear to be partially mediated by involvement in AA and its social support networks, which may serve as a protective factor against relapses to drinking.

Despite evidence for modest effects of specific treatment modalities on alternative measures of drinking behavior, there was no evidence that the different treatments differentially affected the secondary outcomes, such as Depression, Alcohol-related Consequences, or Social Functioning. These findings are highly consistent with the results presented in Chapters 7 and 8. Although Project MATCH did not include an untreated control group, the results suggest that individually delivered psychosocial treatments based on very different treatment philosophies appear to produce comparably good outcomes (Lambert & Bergin, 1994; Hester & Miller, 1995).

Other findings reported in this chapter concern the relationship between post-treatment drinking and various measures of outcome status. In general, the higher the level of post-treatment alcohol consumption, the less the client improved in terms of Alcohol-related Consequences, Depression, Social Functioning, Drug Use, and Days Working (in the Outpatient sample only). This association between post-treatment drinking and the experience of negative outcomes in a variety of life areas supports the notion that treatment-related changes in drinking may have general effects on an individual's overall well-being.

Differences between Outpatient and Aftercare groups

As noted in Chapter 8, there were consistent differences between the Outpatient and Aftercare groups on primary outcome measures of drinking. In general, Aftercare clients showed greater reductions in the frequency and intensity of alcohol consumption as compared with Outpatient clients during the follow-up period. This finding is consistent with a meta-analysis of 100 alcohol treatment outcome studies (published between 1980 and 1992) suggesting that more intensive treatments produced greater abstinence than less intensive treatments (Monahan & Finney, 1996). One explanation for this finding relates to the concept of 'hitting bottom.' That is, Aftercare clients (who presented with more severe alcohol dependence, more alcohol-related problems, and more difficulties in other areas of life functioning) were more likely to avail themselves of treatment and were ready to engage in a change process which involved significant reductions in alcohol consumption. Therefore, they may have begun treatment in Project MATCH in a different phase of their lives in terms of their own readiness to change as compared with the Outpatient group, who may have been experiencing fewer problems related to their drinking and thus had less motivation to make dramatic changes.

However, selection factors may also have been responsible for these differences. Clients were not randomly assigned to Aftercare or to

Outpatient treatment settings. Rather, they were recruited because they either presented for outpatient treatment or had completed inpatient treatment. The ability of Aftercare participants to complete inpatient treatment may have been a selection factor for clients with favorable outcomes, suggesting the presence of capacities such as motivation, self-efficacy, and persistence, which are linked to greater improvement. Finally, given the emphasis on Twelve Step program involvement often communicated through inpatient treatment programs, it may be that Aftercare clients showed greater improvement because of their participation in AA. This would be consistent with a study demonstrating increased sobriety among alcoholics who attended AA after treatment as compared with nonattenders (Hoffmann & Miller, 1992). In this study, the greatest sustained improvement was demonstrated by those individuals who attended AA weekly and went to an aftercare program.

Summary and conclusions

The findings presented in this chapter relating to alternative measures of drinking are highly consistent with the results presented in earlier chapters pertaining to the two primary outcome measures, PDA and DDD. In addition, the same pattern of changes was observed on secondary outcome measures following the initiation of treatment, with both Outpatient clients and Aftercare participants showing large improvements in a variety of different life areas that were maintained throughout the entire follow-up period. Finally, the results suggest that the amount per occasion of drinking affects the resolution of alcohol-related consequences. Greater reductions in drinking seem to forecast improvements in other life areas, suggesting an overall consolidation of treatment benefits that extends beyond a narrow focus on drinking reductions alone.

10

A look inside treatment: therapist effects, the therapeutic alliance, and the process of intentional behavior change

CARLO C. DICLEMENTE, KATHLEEN M. CARROLL,
WILLIAM R. MILLER, GERARD J. CONNORS,
AND DENNIS M. DONOVAN

Therapy is a dynamic interaction among client, therapist, type of treatment, and the process of intentional behavior change. This chapter describes how these different aspects of therapy influenced treatment outcomes. Analyses of client predictors, therapist effects, and specific aspects of treatment lead to the following conclusions: (1) the client's motivation and self-efficacy prior to treatment were the most powerful predictors of post-treatment drinking; (2) with the exception of a few notable outliers, therapists within the three treatments produced similar retention in treatment and comparable drinking outcomes; and (3) the three Project MATCH treatments, despite their differences in philosophy and strategies, affected clients' attitudes and coping activities in remarkably similar ways.

Treatment dimensions and the process of behavior change

Psychosocial treatment for addictive behaviors is dynamic in nature. Evaluations that concentrate solely on outcome cannot completely elucidate the nature of these treatments. Therapy is not static, nor does it produce uniform effects for all clients (Kiesler, 1966). Therapists recognize that clients are a heterogeneous group of individuals who enter treatment with different problems, who experience therapy differently, and who make changes at different rates and in different ways. Clinical trials attempt to distribute this client heterogeneity across treatments in a random fashion, hoping to neutralize the impact of these client differences on treatment compliance and outcomes. Therapist manuals serve to standardize the treatments in order to provide similar experiences for all clients (Donovan et al., 1994; Carroll et al., 1998). The use of detailed

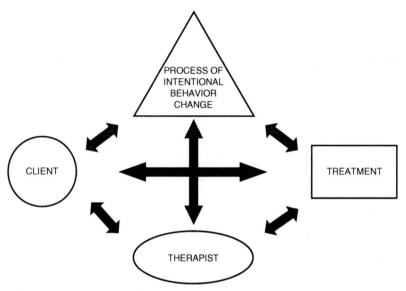

Figure 10.1 Reciprocal influences in the interactions among the critical elements in psychotherapy and behavioral change.

treatment manuals ensures that therapists deliver one and only one of the treatments in as competent and consistent a manner as possible (Waskow, 1984; Donovan & Mattson, 1994). Therapist training and supervision reduce variability in treatment delivery and increase the quality of treatment. In these ways, clinical research seeks to reduce 'noise' variance in treatment implementation and to produce an evaluation of treatment outcome that is valid, generalizable to other treatment settings, and repeatable in other trials.

Nevertheless, the interaction between treatment and client is complex and often eludes our best attempts at standardization. Clinicians and researchers often assert that they are tailoring or matching treatments to clients. Figure 10.1 illustrates the multiple components and the complex interactive nature of the treatment matching concept. In addition, each component has multiple dimensions. Treatments can be characterized in terms of their philosophy, techniques, intensity, and duration. Therapists differ in personal characteristics, beliefs, training, and skills. The client brings to this interaction personal characteristics, beliefs, skills, and prior experience. Finally, there is the dynamic process of intentional behavioral change that is characterized by motivation, coping activities, and expectancies about change. Every attempt to examine treatment outcome is really an attempt to understand the interactions among the treatment, the therapist, the client, and the process of intentional behavior change.

The impact of these components on one another is reciprocal in nature (DiClemente & Scott, 1997), as illustrated by the double-sided arrows in the figure. Therapists can enhance or interfere with the client's process of behavioral change; interventions can do the same (DiClemente et al., 1992). Clients can refuse to engage in the behavioral change process and can sabotage the treatment, or they can comply with the therapy, but remain ambivalent about it and refuse to change. Interventions can be matched or mismatched either to the characteristics of the client or to the intricacies of the process of intentional behavioral change. Therapists and clients can be matched or mismatched in terms of gender, personal characteristics, styles, or goals (Beutler et al., 1994).

There is a rich tradition in the psychotherapy literature that emphasizes the importance of envisioning therapy not simply as a uniform 'black box' that patients pass through in similar ways (Sloane et al., 1975; Elkin et al., 1989). Treatment outcomes are affected by the implementation of the treatment, engagement in treatment, and client satisfaction with treatment (Bergin & Garfield, 1994). In addition, there is an extensive literature on how therapist characteristics, the nature of the therapeutic relationship, and environmental influences affect treatment outcomes (Luborsky et al., 1975; Bergin & Garfield, 1994). More recently, psychotherapy research has begun to evaluate how changes in the cognitive and behavioral coping activities engendered by therapy interact with treatment outcome (Goldfried, 1980; Prochaska et al., 1992). Despite the extensive effort dedicated to these endeavors, we still do not understand how therapy works, what the unique and common dimensions of effective treatments are, and how treatments initiate or interact with the individual client's process of intentional behavioral change (Lindström, 1992).

In addition to these efforts to understand treatments, there has been a growing body of literature dedicated to understanding the process of intentional behavior change as it occurs both within and outside of treatment, particularly in the area of addictive behaviors (Tuchfield, 1981; Moos et al., 1990; Prochaska & DiClemente, 1992; Prochaska et al., 1992; Miller et al., 1993; Valliant, 1995; Sobell et al., 1996; Sobell & Sobell, 1998). Measures of decisional considerations, processes of change, self-efficacy, and motivational stages of change have been developed to clarify what happens during successful cessation or modification of alcohol and drug use. By separating client characteristics and formal treatment from the process of intentional change for specific behaviors, researchers have begun to isolate change principles that can be examined across treatments and problem behaviors (Goldfried, 1980; DiClemente & Prochaska, 1998).

Using pre-treatment, during-treatment and post-treatment assessment batteries, Project MATCH investigators were able to assess not only relevant client characteristics and drinking outcomes, but also therapy dimensions and behavioral change dimensions typically not evaluated in previous research with alcohol-dependent populations (DiClemente et al., 1994b). Moreover, the large number of therapists included in this trial permitted a more systematic examination of therapist characteristics (Project MATCH Research Group, 1998b, 1998c). This chapter describes what was learned about the therapies, the therapists, and the clients, and how these factors interacted with the process of intentional behavior change.

The treatments

The rationales for the three treatments studied in Project MATCH are fully described in Chapter 4. The basic assumption underlying the choice of treatments was that Cognitive–Behavioral Therapy (CBT), Motivational Enhancement Therapy (MET) and Twelve Step Facilitation (TSF) differed sufficiently in philosophy, emphasis, mechanisms of action, and techniques, and that these elements would produce different matching effects. Each of the treatments was intended to be powerful enough to produce a significant modification of drinking behavior. Moreover, the investigators intended the treatments to be equally effective, because superiority of one treatment would have made matching effects more difficult to detect (Longabaugh & Wirtz, 2001). For example, if CBT were better overall for all clients, matching some clients to a less effective treatment would be inadvisable.

As described in Chapter 4, the three treatments were different from each other. Independent ratings of videotapes of over 1200 treatment sessions demonstrated clear differences among treatments on basic elements outlined in the therapy manuals (Carroll et al., 1998). CBT therapists assigned homework, focused on drinking cues, and conducted skills training. TSF therapists talked about the Twelve Steps, encouraged Alcoholics Anonymous (AA) attendance, and focused on denial. MET therapists gave specific feedback about drinking problems and focused on clarifying the client's goals. Figure 10.2 illustrates differences among the three therapies in treatment-specific techniques rated by independent observers.

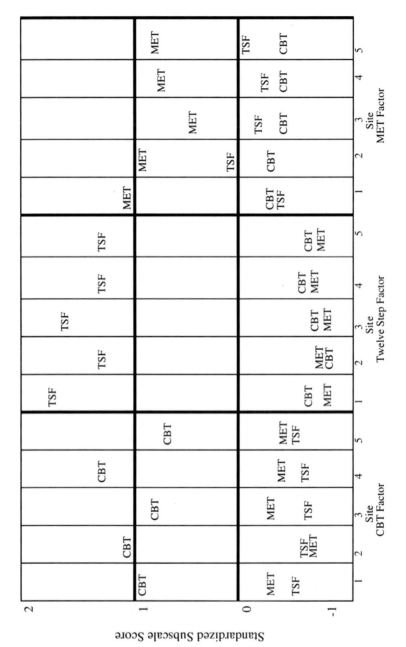

Figure 10.2 Treatment discriminability, Outpatient study Treatment subscale standardized scores by Treatment Condition and Site.

MET was designed to be a briefer treatment, consisting of only four sessions, in contrast to the 12 sessions of both CBT and TSF. As expected, MET clients attended fewer sessions of treatment and thus had less contact with the therapists (Carroll et al., 1998; Mattson et al., 1998). However, MET clients attended the final session more often than their counterparts in the other treatments. Although the final session was scheduled 6 weeks after the third session, the large majority of MET clients came to that final session. Thus, the trial successfully produced the desired contrast in the intensity of the treatments but kept them equivalent in extensiveness over time.

TSF was designed to assist clients to begin working the Twelve Steps and to initiate or continue attendance at AA meetings. TSF clients went to significantly more AA meetings during treatment than clients in the other two conditions (Carroll et al., 1998). AA attendance was higher for TSF clients even in the Aftercare arm of the trial, in which clients in all three treatments were encouraged to attend AA meetings during the residential care they received before beginning the Project MATCH Aftercare treatment. Thus, the TSF treatment engaged clients in significantly more AA attendance.

The sharp discriminability of the treatments stands in marked contrast to the other findings of Project MATCH. Treatment differences were minimal on most measures of drinking outcomes and elements of behavior change (Chapters 7, 8, and 9). Other studies have reported similar findings of comparable outcomes for distinctive treatments (Elkin et al., 1989; Ouimette et al., 1997). Similar effects produced by different treatments can be explained in several ways: (1) common elements of the treatments produce similar changes; (2) the treatments represent different paths to achieving the same end; (3) there is a common process of individual behavior change that is facilitated equally well by the different treatments; or (4) the treatments have no effect in producing the outcomes. These explanations are considered further as other active ingredients of treatment and dimensions of behavioral change of the trial are explored.

The therapists

Therapists in Project MATCH were chosen to be typical of the therapists who conduct these three treatments in the 'real' world. Therapists were 'nested' or grouped within treatments rather than randomly assigned to treatments. A total of 80 therapists (26 in CBT, 26 in MET, and 28 in TSF) were certified to treat Project MATCH clients (Project MATCH Research Group, 1998b). The TSF therapists differed in expected ways from those in the other two conditions. TSF therapists had fewer years of formal education. They were also more likely to have had alcohol problems themselves, to be certified alcohol and drug counselors, to endorse a disease model of alcohol problems, and to make choices based on personal values and subjective concerns. On the other hand, there were no differences across treatments in therapists' duration of employment in the field, gender distribution, and basic personality dimensions as measured by the Edwards Personal Preference Scales.

As in other studies of therapist effects, there were significant differences among therapists in their clients' drinking outcomes (Project MATCH Research Group, 1998d). However, these differences were generally accounted for by a single therapist whose clients fared significantly *worse* in terms of drinking either during treatment or during the follow-up period. In these analyses, different individual therapists represented an 'outlier' for each of the different outcomes so that there was no single 'bad' therapist. When each outlier was removed from the analysis, therapist differences in outcomes disappeared in all but one case (MET, Aftercare arm). Thus, there were comparatively few outcome differences among therapists. This suggests that training may have been helpful in reducing performance variability among therapists.

Treatment outcomes were related to several therapist characteristics (Project MATCH Research Group, 1998d). However, these attributes showed a variable pattern of relationship to client outcomes across treatment and time. For example, the therapist's level of education and years of experience had little impact in CBT and MET, but were negatively related to TSF outcomes. There was one interesting therapist matching effect, with the female Outpatient clients having better drinking outcomes with female therapists. This finding must be considered tentative because the overall gender by treatment matching hypothesis was not supported.

A few differences were found among therapists in other aspects of the therapy evaluations. MET Outpatient therapists differed on ratings of the Working Alliance provided by the client. However, there were no significant differences in retention among the therapists. Reports of client satisfaction differed by therapist (Project MATCH Research Group, 1998b). In fact, client satisfaction varied significantly across therapists for all three treatments in both arms of the trial. These differences, nevertheless, offer little assistance in explaining similarities or differences in drinking outcomes across treatments. The greatest differences among the therapists and the largest number of associations between therapist characteristics and client outcomes occurred with the TSF therapists. However, the TSF treatments produced comparable and, at times, slightly better abstinence outcomes during the post-treatment period.

Contrary to clinical wisdom, the therapist's recovery status, age, and beliefs about alcohol problems did not emerge as significant outcome predictors in the different treatments. However, it must be noted again that most of these analyses were done within treatments because therapists were nested within therapies. If therapists had been randomly assigned to different treatments, the results might have been different.

Therapist characteristics have been suggested as a promising but largely unstudied influence that can affect treatment outcome (Luborsky et al., 1985; Crits-Christoph et al., 1990; Beutler et al., 1994; Najavits & Weiss, 1994). Examination of the therapists in Project MATCH indicates that there were some therapists and therapist characteristics that were related both to treatment satisfaction and to drinking outcomes. However, no clear picture emerged of the critical therapist attributes or beliefs that produced consistently positive or negative outcomes. In many ways, this may be due to the fact that Project MATCH mostly recruited seasoned therapists who were committed to the treatments they delivered, and who were trained and closely supervised to improve their competence and adherence to detailed treatment manuals. Although there was clear diversity among the therapists and differences in their delivery of the treatments, with the exception of a few notable outliers, therapists within the three treatments produced similar retention in treatment and comparable drinking outcomes.

The working alliance

Another area where speculation suggests that treatment outcomes can be influenced is in the nature of the client–therapist relationship. Some theorists, like Carl Rogers (1957), believe that this relationship is the primary curative factor in psychotherapy. Much of the research spawned by Rogers and his colleagues has focused on therapist qualities of warmth, empathy, and genuineness as critical elements in the process of change (Truax & Carkuff, 1967). However, the focus has shifted more recently to the interaction between therapist and client, often referred to as the therapeutic or working alliance (Horvath & Greenberg, 1994). Research

Table 10.1. *Sample items from the client version of the Working Alliance Inventory*

---

1. What I am doing in therapy gives me new ways to look at my problems
2. (Therapist) does not understand what I am trying to accomplish in therapy
3. I am frustrated by what is going on in therapy
4. (Therapist) and I trust one another
5. (Therapist) and I have different ideas about what my problems are
6. (Therapist) and I are working toward mutually agreed-upon goals
7. My relationship with (therapist) is very important to me
8. I am confident in (therapist)'s ability to help me

(Horvath & Symonds, 1991) has found a moderate but consistent relationship between the therapeutic alliance and treatment outcome across several types of therapy (e.g., psychodynamic, cognitive, eclectic). Meta-analyses have supported the importance of the working alliance, particularly in the early stages of treatment (Luborsky et al., 1985; Horvath & Symonds, 1991; Krupnick et al., 1996; Luborsky et al., 1997).

In Project MATCH, we evaluated the relationship between therapist and client using the Working Alliance Inventory (WAI; Connors et al., 1997). Both the client and the therapist rated the alliance after the second treatment session. Therapists also provided ratings later in the treatment. Table 10.1 provides some examples of the WAI items. WAI total scores, whether provided by the client or by the therapist in the Outpatient arm of the trial, were significant predictors of treatment participation and of the frequency and intensity of drinking, both during the treatment period and during the post-treatment follow-up. In the Aftercare arm, the WAI demonstrated much less predictive ability. Aftercare therapists' ratings of the working alliance predicted only the percentage of days abstinent during treatment and during the post-treatment period (Connors et al., 1997). Thus, for Outpatient clients, the alliance between the therapist and the client was an important factor in successful treatment outcome across all three treatments, a finding consistent with prior research (Horvath & Symonds, 1991; Horvath & Greenberg, 1994). Moreover, WAI ratings by clients and therapists were not highly correlated. Client ratings were stronger predictors of treatment participation and outcome than were ratings provided by the therapists.

The lack of a stronger effect for the Working Alliance variable in the

Aftercare arm is understandable. Because these clients had received more intensive treatment prior to entry into Project MATCH, they had other therapy relationships that could affect outcome. Moreover, most clients began the Aftercare treatment abstinent. The second session of the After-care treatment may have been too early for the client to accurately evaluate the treatment relationship in terms of how helpful it would be in sustaining abstinence. The Outpatient relationships between alliance and outcomes probably provide a better test of the influence of the therapeutic relationship on drinking outcomes.

Although not reported in prior research, the Working Alliance was related to client Motivational Readiness to Change. In the Outpatient arm of the trial, Motivation as well as the Working Alliance predicted drinking outcomes (Connors et al., 1997; Project MATCH Research Group, 1997a). Several analyses were conducted to examine the impact of pre-treatment Motivation on WAI ratings provided by the client and therapist (measured at session 2). Motivation was significantly and positively related to client ratings of the Working Alliance in both arms of the trial (Connors et al., 2000; DiClemente et al., 2001b). Motivation was the single largest predictor of these WAI ratings in both arms, although there were other predictors as well (Connors et al., 2000). The more motivated the client, the higher the ratings of the Working Alliance with the therapist. The positive influence of client motivation on therapeutic alliance ratings was supported in other analyses, which demonstrated that client readiness to change moderates the relationship between the alliance and drinking outcomes. More motivated clients see therapy and therapists more positively and change their drinking behavior more than those who are less motivated. This latter effect is true only for those clients in the Outpatient condition.

The analyses of the Working Alliance support a role for the relationship between the therapist and the client in the process of change. The most important perspective on this relationship appeared to be that of the client. These relationships between alliance and outcome were most clear in the Outpatient condition, where the Project MATCH therapist played a more prominent role in the clients' treatment. However, this relationship was intimately connected to the location of the client in the intentional process of behavior change as the more motivated clients rated the alliance higher (DiClemente et al., 2001a).

Client satisfaction with treatment

At the end of treatment, clients were asked how satisfied they were with their therapist, the number of sessions, the overall treatment, and the extent to which the treatment met their needs (Donovan et al., in press). Clients were also asked how much they had changed since beginning treatment. Several important findings emerged from these analyses. Client satisfaction with treatment was modestly related to perceived changes during treatment ($r = 0.38$). Client overall satisfaction was similarly correlated ($r = 0.43$) with client ratings of the helpfulness of the various elements of treatment (i.e., learning skills, telling problems to someone, getting feedback on alcohol use).

Although clients reported a high degree of satisfaction with all three of the Project MATCH therapies, meaningful differences were found between the two study arms. Clients in Aftercare were more satisfied with their treatment experiences than were those in Outpatient treatment. Aftercare clients had higher levels of satisfaction with treatment, were more satisfied with their therapists and with the number of therapy sessions received, and were more willing to return to the therapy again if they needed help in the future. Nevertheless, across both arms of the trial, there were few differences in client satisfaction among the three Project MATCH treatments. Outpatient clients in MET were less satisfied with their treatment compared to those in CBT and TSF. This was probably due to the smaller number of sessions delivered in MET and to the fact that, during treatment, the clients were drinking slightly more than the participants in the other two treatments. Clients who received MET and TSF as Outpatients were less satisfied with the number of sessions and with their overall treatment compared to the clients who received MET and TSF in Aftercare (Donovan et al., in press).

As expected, greater treatment attendance was positively associated with client satisfaction, at least among the Outpatient clients. Completion of the TSF and CBT treatments was associated with higher levels of satisfaction, but this relationship was not found for MET clients. However, across all three treatments, the total number of weeks in therapy was significantly related to general satisfaction, perceived helpfulness of the therapy, and perceived improvement in drinking status.

Interestingly, there was no significant relationship between client ratings of the Working Alliance and client general satisfaction in either the Outpatient or Aftercare arms of the trial. Although client evaluations of the

Working Alliance at the second therapy session were positively related to drinking outcomes, these ratings were not related to satisfaction with therapy at the end of treatment. In contrast, in the Aftercare arm there were several significant negative correlations between therapist WAI ratings and client general satisfaction at the end of treatment. Thus, for Aftercare clients, the more positively the therapist evaluated the alliance, the less satisfied were the clients.

Satisfaction with treatment, however, was strongly related to changes in drinking over the course of treatment. Individuals with fewer days abstinent and with more Drinks per Drinking Day (DDA) during treatment were significantly less satisfied overall. They also perceived the therapeutic process as less helpful to them, and perceived themselves as having changed less than those with lower levels of drinking. What was true for drinking during treatment also held for post-treatment improvement. Clients whose status at the end of treatment was improved from baseline were significantly more satisfied than those whose outcome was poor, reflecting little or no change from baseline (Donovan et al., in press). Success and satisfaction went hand in hand. Satisfaction differed by setting, as did success. However, there were few differences by treatment condition. For the most part, satisfaction seemed related to drinking behavior change but not to specific treatments.

The process of intentional behavioral change

Dimensions of the process of behavioral change were assessed at baseline, during treatment, and at post-treatment. Client Motivation, Alcohol Abstinence Self-efficacy, and vulnerability to relapse (assessed as Temptation to drink) were measured at baseline. During treatment, clients completed session reports that monitored coping mechanisms (processes of change), difficulty with not drinking, and perceived ability (efficacy) to abstain. At the end of treatment, experiential and behavioral processes of change, Alcohol Abstinence Self-efficacy, Motivation, and drinking outcome variables were again assessed. These measures were used to monitor the process of intentional behavioral change during and after treatment.

As previously reported (Project MATCH Research Group, 1997a, 1997b, 1998a), client Motivation predicted drinking outcomes for Outpatients throughout the follow-up period. How motivated individuals were to change their drinking as they entered treatment was a potent indicator of long-term success among Outpatients. This relationship was not found for the Aftercare clients. However, in both arms of the trial, Motivation showed little interaction with the three treatments, suggesting that, for the most part, Motivation functioned similarly across treatments. There was a brief period of time immediately after the conclusion of treatment when CBT was associated with better drinking outcomes for less motivated Outpatients. At the end of the 1-year follow-up period, less motivated clients in MET drank significantly less than CBT clients, as hypothesized. However, both of these effects on drinking were ephemeral (Project MATCH Research Group, 1997a).

Contrary to what has been found in other trials, the client's motivation to change did not predict treatment attendance (Smith et al., 1995; Mattson et al., 1998). The high level of treatment attendance in Project MATCH appears unrelated to motivation to change drinking behavior and to be more a function of extrinsic motivation, the structure of the treatments, and the strategies used for treatment compliance (Kabela & Kadden, 1997).

Motivation to change drinking was not highly correlated with other client characteristics. Motivation tends to be a changeable psychological state, unlike more stable characteristics, such as sociopathy, gender, and alcoholic subtype. Motivation was positively correlated with Alcohol Dependence ($r = 0.25$) as well as with prior AA Involvement ($r = 0.18$), and negatively correlated with social functioning ($r = -0.20$). There was a moderate positive correlation between motivation and measures of drinking consequences and distress. Clearly, there was a relationship between initial Motivation and acknowledgment of consequences and problems with drinking. However, the sheer number of consequences does not account for all motivation to change, as the 'hitting bottom' view of motivation would propose. In fact, the relationship is small. We did find that the more clients acknowledged problems, the more ready they were to change drinking behavior. Clinicians who view the client's acknowledgment of the connection between the drinking and the consequences as an indicator of motivation at intake to treatment have been looking in the right direction. However, Motivation was unrelated to most other measures of client characteristics, like Sociopathy, Psychopathology, Religiosity, and Cognitive Impairment.

Motivation was also related to other client process of change variables. As noted above, in both arms of the trial, motivation to change predicted a positive Working Alliance between the client and the therapist. Motivation also predicted use of experiential and behavioral processes of change both

Table 10.2. *Sample items from the experiential and behavioral processes of Change scale*

Experiential Processes of Change
1. I get upset when I think about illnesses caused by my drinking
2. I stop to think that my drinking is causing problems for other people
3. I become disappointed with myself when I depend on alcohol

Behavioral Processes of Change
1. I do something else instead of drinking to deal with tension
2. I make commitments to myself not to drink
3. I avoid situations that encourage me to drink

---

during treatment (at the second session) and at the end of treatment (DiClemente et al., 2001b). In general, Motivation to change drinking was related to engagement with the therapist in treatment and to the coping activities that clients used to stop drinking and to remain abstinent. Motivation at entry to treatment was also significantly related to attendance at AA meetings during treatment, particularly for the TSF clients ($r = 0.18$ for Outpatient and $r = 0.13$ for Aftercare clients). Motivation appeared to be related to how individuals engaged with the therapist and how active they were in using cognitive and behavioral coping skills and external resources to modify their drinking.

One of the interesting findings of these analyses involved the client's experiential and behavioral processes of change. These processes represent the coping activities identified by different systems of psychotherapy (Prochaska & DiClemente, 1984; Prochaska et al., 1992; DiClemente & Prochaska, 1998). In previous research, ten processes have been identified that fall into two broad categories: cognitive/experiential processes and behavioral processes (DiClemente & Prochaska, 1998). In Project MATCH, these ten processes were assessed after each therapy session and at post-treatment follow-up. Clients were asked how often each of these activities or experiences had occurred recently or during the past week. Table 10.2 gives sample items for both the experiential and the behavioral processes of change. Individuals who attended different treatments in Project MATCH reported remarkably similar process activity both during treatment and at the post-treatment assessment. Coping activities measured by the processes of change did not differ across treatments or interact with treatment except in a few cases (DiClemente et al., 2001b). However, reported change activities during treatment and at post-treatment, particularly behavioral process activity, predicted drinking outcomes (Carbonari & DiClemente, 2000). Although philosophically distinct and objectively discriminable, the three treatments were related to clients' coping activities to manage their drinking in the same way, because there were no interactions or differences among the treatments on these processes of change.

The picture for Alcohol Abstinence Self-efficacy was similar to the one for motivation. Self-efficacy (confidence) at baseline for Outpatients was a significant predictor of drinking – Percent Days Abstinent (PDA) and DDD – during the post-treatment period, even as far as the 3-year follow-up. Interestingly, Self-efficacy and Motivation were not correlated at pretreatment ($r = 0.01$, Outpatient, $r = 0.08$, Aftercare). Thus, they appear to be independent dimensions of the client process of behavior change. Clients entering Aftercare from a more intensive treatment setting reported more abstinence and more self-efficacy to abstain from drinking during the MATCH treatments, as would be expected. However, Self-efficacy increased during treatment for both Outpatients and Aftercare clients and leveled off during the follow-up period. Self-efficacy both reflects and predicts drinking behavior (DiClemente et al., 2001a). These findings support the interactive nature of the cognitive and behavioral aspects of the client change process, as described by Bandura (1986).

There was some evidence that self-efficacy interacted with treatments in the Aftercare arm of the trial. As hypothesized, low Self-efficacy CBT clients had better drinking outcomes than low Self-efficacy MET clients (Project MATCH Research Group, 1997b). However, the interaction was limited to drinking outcomes during the treatment period. Alcohol Abstinence Self-efficacy at the end of treatment did not differ by treatment. Once again, these data indicate that the treatments either interacted with or failed to interact with the client process of intentional behavioral change in similar ways. CBT and MET, which targeted self-efficacy in their treatment strategies, did not produce significantly different levels of Alcohol Abstinence Self-efficacy at the end of treatment in comparison with TSF, which ostensibly asked clients to admit powerlessness over drinking. For all clients, Self-efficacy assessed at the end of treatment was a better predictor of future drinking than was pre-treatment Self-efficacy. Client evaluations of the Temptation to drink in 20 high-risk situations were also strong predictors of drinking after treatment (DiClemente et al., 2001a).

Indicators of the process of intentional behavioral change (Self-efficacy, experiential and behavioral coping activities, and Motivation) varied over the course of treatment and were significantly related to the changes in drinking behavior throughout the year-long follow-up period (Carbonari & DiClemente, 2000). Their ability to predict drinking frequency and intensity extends to the 3-year follow-up for the Outpatient clients (the only cohort followed that long). Pre-treatment values of these measures showed a greater relationship to future drinking in the Outpatient arm compared to the Aftercare arm. Client indicators of engagement in the process of behavioral change shifted over the course of treatment, as did their drinking (e.g., Self-efficacy increased and Temptation decreased). However, these indicators showed little interaction with specific treatments. Because of the absence of an untreated control group, it was impossible to determine the effect of treatment on the client's process of change. However, the analyses indicated that many cognitive and behavioral coping activities as well as client attitudes changed from the beginning to the end of treatment and that the treatments did not differentially affect this process in any significant manner (Carbonari & DiClemente, 2000).

Conclusions

If we examine the interactions between client characteristics and client intentional behavioral change variables, on the one hand, and the treatments and therapists, on the other, the process findings from Project MATCH point to several interesting conclusions.

First, the client's self-evaluations were the most predictive variables among those assessed in Project MATCH. Motivation and Self-efficacy assessed at baseline were the most potent predictors of drinking following the end of treatment for Outpatients. Clients' evaluations of the Working Alliance predicted drinking better than therapist reports. Clients' reports of experiential and behavioral activities designed to cope with changes in drinking behavior predicted future drinking better than treatment condition and objective ratings of within-treatment activities. Although client self-assessments are subject to social desirability bias and dissimulation, and can vary by setting (Outpatient versus Aftercare), asking clear questions about salient issues and events increases the accuracy of these reports (Babor et al., 1990; Schwarz, 1999). The central role of the client in changing drinking behavior within the therapy enterprise was highlighted in our analyses of the various dimensions of treatment and the process of intentional behavior change.

Measured at entry into treatment, during treatment, and at the end of treatment, these self-evaluations interacted with changes in drinking behavior and predicted successful and unsuccessful drinking outcomes. Markers of the intentional behavioral change process were affected in similar ways by the three treatments. More importantly, some behavioral change markers, such as Motivation to Change, influenced other important treatment process variables, such as the Working Alliance between therapist and client, as rated by the client (Connors et al., 2000).

A second conclusion is that when trained, supervised, and monitored to deliver manual-guided treatments, therapists appear to be more alike than different in the skillfulness and fidelity with which they deliver individual therapies. As described in Chapter 4, discriminability ratings indicated that the 80 therapists delivered each of the treatments faithfully. Across multiple treatment sites, the Project MATCH therapists demonstrated little variability in delivery of the treatments. However, despite our best attempts at standardization, individual therapists could interfere with or potentiate the client's drinking behavior change. At least one 'outlier' therapist in each of the treatment conditions produced poorer drinking outcomes for their clients, which set them apart from the other therapists who were offering the same treatment. Therapists played an important role in the interaction with clients in treatment. There emerged, however, no clear picture of what attributes or skills were critical influences on drinking behavior. The lack of sizable outcome differences between treatments and the lack of differences in client and therapist ratings of the Working Alliance showed that, when they practice different manually driven treatments, therapists are more alike than different in how they interact with the client.

A third conclusion is that treatments that differ substantially in philosophy and in strategies produce similar outcomes and affect clients in similar ways. It was not completely clear from our analyses whether the common elements of the treatments accounted for the homogeneous impact on the client or whether there were different, equally effective strategies that produced the similarities in process measures and drinking outcomes. TSF clients, for example, did take a different route to abstinence by attending significantly more AA meetings, yet CBT and MET clients had similar outcomes. The matching effects that are reported in other chapters of this volume (Chapters 7 and 8) also suggest differential pathways for a similar process of behavioral change. The absence of a control group did not allow us to establish the critical differences in process activity and outcomes that would empirically support the role of treatment. However, there was a significant amount of sustained change over time that differed significantly from the clients' reported drinking history prior to entering these treatments. Something happened coinciding with, if not caused by, participation in a Project MATCH treatment. One interpretation of these findings is that the observed changes were largely client driven and unrelated to the treatments. Without a control group, this interpretation cannot be refuted. However, prior large-scale studies that have employed a true control group and several active treatments have found superior effects for treated groups, even if they found no differences between the active treatments (Sloane et al., 1975; Elkin et al., 1989; Bergin & Garfield, 1994).

This analysis of Project MATCH data offers interesting information about treatment process and outcome. Some findings confirm prior research, whereas some challenge current assumptions. It is hoped that these findings will encourage new initiatives examining therapists, the working alliance, and diverse treatments, as well as the role of intentional behavioral change processes and dimensions in both psychosocial and pharmacotherapy treatments for alcohol and other problems. The interactions among the client, the process of intentional behavioral change, the therapist, and the treatment are complex. Although we cannot definitively answer the question of how these different treatments produced similar outcomes, the Project MATCH process data support a common process of behavioral change, with the treatments providing different paths to achieving the same coping activities and drinking outcomes. There may be 'different strokes for different folks,' but they all seem to be swimming in the same river. As is often the case, our process research has answered some questions but has also raised more interesting ones.

11

Participation and involvement in Alcoholics Anonymous

J. SCOTT TONIGAN, GERARD J. CONNORS,
AND WILLIAM R. MILLER

Despite being the largest mutual-help organization for alcoholics in the world, Alcoholics Anonymous (AA) has rarely been investigated with the kind of rigorous methodological attention it received in Project MATCH. This chapter describes the patterns of AA utilization, the relationship between AA participation and abstinence, and the benefits associated with AA participation. As expected, Twelve Step Facilitation (TSF) therapy was associated with increased AA attendance, which in turn was associated with increased abstinence. The findings highlight the importance of initiating AA attendance during formal treatment, provide compelling evidence for the value of AA as an adjunct to professional treatment, and suggest practical ways to maximize the potential benefits of AA through TSF.

A mutual-help program is a group of individuals who possess a common problem, who seek relief from the problem using a common plan, and who are not led by a professional. Alcoholics Anonymous (AA) originated in 1933 and has grown to become the largest and most popular mutual-help program for people with alcohol-related problems. Annually, it is estimated that 3.5 million people attend an AA meeting (Room, 1993) and there are about 96 000 different meeting locations (Alcoholics Anonymous, 1997). The curative plan of AA is embodied in the Twelve Steps and, with the aid of a more experienced member, or 'sponsor', AA members sequentially 'work' each of the Twelve Steps. As described in the AA core literature, alcohol-related problems are a three-fold malady consisting of spiritual, mental, and physical aspects, and relief from this malady comes with working the steps (Alcoholics Anonymous, 1976, 1981).

AA is an abstinence-based program. Alcohol-free living is an explicit goal, but abstinence from illicit mood-altering drugs is also strongly advocated. It is important to observe that lifelong abstinence is viewed in AA in the context of living one day at a time. Considerable tolerance is found in AA regarding members who continue or return to drinking. The third tradition of AA states that the only requirement for AA membership is a *desire* to stop drinking, and failed efforts to achieve or maintain abstinence are accepted with the provision that AA meetings are not disrupted by intoxicated persons. AA members make an important distinction between abstinence and sobriety, with sobriety being the loftier goal. Within the AA culture, abstinence refers strictly to the cessation of alcohol use, whereas sobriety refers to both abstinence and the successful incorporation of Twelve Step principles into one's daily life. Although Project MATCH was not a study of the effectiveness of AA, the large and diverse samples in the study nevertheless provided a unique opportunity to examine AA attendance and involvement after formal treatment, as well as AA participation for those clients receiving therapy that included encouragement to affiliate with AA in particular.

Prior research on Alcoholics Anonymous

Reviews of the empirical research on AA have concluded that drinking and problem severity are positively predictive of subsequent AA affiliation, and that AA attendance is modestly associated with improved functioning and abstinence (Emrick et al., 1993; Tonigan et al., 1996b; Emrick, 1999). Reviewers note, however, that these conclusions are based mostly upon single-group studies that did not use rigorous scientific methods (Tonigan et al., 1996b). Studies employing more rigorous methods have indicated that commitment to abstinence, primary appraisal of the problem (Morgenstern et al., 1997), and problem severity (e.g., in substance use, family functioning, and psychological status) predict AA affiliation (Humphreys et al., 1991).

Little attention has been paid to understanding how formal treatment may *facilitate* AA utilization. This lack of attention has led to uncertainty about which aspects of AA ideology and practices ought to be encouraged in formal treatment, and how such aspects may predict sustained involvement in AA. Traditionally, encouragement to attend AA by treatment providers is just that, required AA meeting attendance. The expectation is that clients will continue attending AA after treatment. The underlying assumption is that attendance begets commitment. Commitment to the practices of AA, in turn, is felt to predict sustained membership. AA meeting attendance, however, is only one dimension of the AA experience.

Other dimensions include practicing prescribed AA behaviors, such as working the Twelve Steps.

Work by Montgomery et al. (1995) and Snow et al. (1994) questions the logic that AA attendance in itself predicts subsequent commitment to AA practices. Contrary to AA folklore, 'bring the body and the mind will follow' may not always be true (Alcoholics Anonymous, 1981). In particular, Montgomery and colleagues reported only a modest positive association between AA attendance and AA involvement in clients discharged 6 months earlier from an inpatient treatment center. Likewise, only a modest positive correlation between attendance and participation in AA-related activities was found by Snow et al. (1994) in AA members with long-term sobriety.

Recognizing the need for more than just advice to attend AA when sustained participation was desired, two studies evaluated AA practices of clients (after formal treatment) when the treatment included a multi-faceted Twelve Step orientation. In a study of conjoint therapy involving male alcoholics and their nonalcoholic spouses, McCrady et al. (1999) reported that AA attendance could be improved and that an AA sponsor could be found *during* treatment through therapist encouragement. Relative to two therapies not emphasizing AA principles, this AA-focused therapy, however, did not produce proportionately more AA step work or socialization with other AA members. Also important, between-group therapy differences in AA attendance during treatment faded by 6 months after treatment (McCrady et al., 1996).

In a second study involving a Twelve Step-focused formal therapy, Caldwell and Cutter (1998) evaluated the relationships between frequency of AA attendance and 19 prescribed practices that indicate commitment to AA (e.g., declaring a Home Group, becoming active in AA activities, engaging in conversations with AA members both before and after meetings). Three groups of AA affiliates were identified when evaluating the AA attendance patterns for the first 10 weeks after treatment (70 days). Low AA attenders (<20 meetings in 70 days) were significantly less likely to attend meetings that fostered discussion and close relationships. Both mid-level and high-level AA attenders reported significantly greater use of sponsors than low-level attenders, but high-level attenders reported more contact with other AA members than mid-level attenders. Although this study did not include a non-Twelve Step comparison group, it appears, as found by McCrady et al. (1996), that formal treatment can facilitate AA meeting attendance, and that, for reasons that are still unclear, some individuals will also show commitment to AA-related practices. It is important to stress that the directionality of attendance and commitment to AA-related practices was not addressed in these studies.

Measures of AA attendance and commitment were included in the Project MATCH assessment battery for several reasons. First, the Twelve Step Facilitation (TSF) condition was specifically intended to increase affiliation with and involvement in AA (Nowinski et al., 1992). Measurement of Twelve Step participation was thus one of several methods used to assess the fidelity of the TSF protocol. Second, the primary and secondary matching hypotheses (see Chapter 6) did not specify client–AA matching predictions *per se*, but several matching hypotheses included AA participation as a causal mechanism that might explain how client–treatment matching would operate (e.g., Connors et al., 2001; Tonigan et al., 2001). Third, alcohol treatment outcomes are mediated by a number of factors, one of which appears to be AA participation (Emrick et al., 1993; Ouimette et al., 1998; Humphreys et al., 1999). Identification of the relative value of mediators associated with post-treatment functioning thus argued for measurement of AA exposure after formal treatment.

The findings reported in Chapters 7 and 8 that the TSF treatment was as effective as the more empirically supported Cognitive–Behavioral Therapy (CBT) and Motivational Enhancement Therapy (MET), and was actually more effective on selected abstinence-based secondary outcome measures (see Chapter 9), generated additional enthusiasm for understanding the AA experiences reported by the Project MATCH clients. Findings from another large aftercare clinical trial (Ouimette et al., 1997) also suggested that Twelve Step-based therapy was as effective as CBT. Common to these Twelve Step-based therapies was active facilitation into AA.

The purpose of this chapter is to describe the AA experiences reported by Project MATCH clients. Because measurement reliability and validity are essential for theory-driven research on AA, the first section provides test–retest findings and the results of comparing client and collateral reports of client AA attendance. The central question addressed in this section is the accuracy of self-reported AA attendance. The next section of this chapter compares the actual rates of AA attendance and involvement among Project MATCH Outpatient and Aftercare clients. Here we describe the topography of AA attendance and involvement across the follow-up phase of the study. Of substantial clinical importance is the identification of distinct patterns of AA utilization, and how such patterns vary as a function of AA meeting attendance and involvement. We then describe the relationship between AA participation and abstinence, as well as the benefits associated with AA participation.

Measurement issues: reliability and validity

Can clients with alcohol-related problems report on past and current AA exposure reliably and accurately? Reliability refers to *consistency* in measurement of a belief, attitude, or behavior. Error in measurement attenuates estimates of a relationship, with the implication that reliable or consistent measurement is more important when small relationships are anticipated. Validity, on the other hand, refers to the accuracy of what is measured, i.e., whether it actually is what it is believed to be.

Four measures used to assess AA exposure were evaluated for reliability and validity. Each of these measures provided a different perspective of AA participation. Attendance at AA meetings was measured using the Form-90 (Miller, 1996), the central measure of drinking behavior in the study. Commitment to AA practices and beliefs was measured using the Alcoholics Anonymous Involvement scale (AAI; Tonigan et al., 1996a). Finally, two questionnaires provided single items measuring subjective ratings of the helpfulness of AA emphasis during treatment and the usefulness of AA for maintaining sobriety.

Form-90

The Form-90 was administered at intake and at all follow-ups. The frequency of AA meeting attendance (in days) was recorded at each interview. Because the actual number of days included in an assessment window differed from client to client, reported frequency of AA attendance was divided by the total number of days in an assessment interval to derive the percentage of days of AA attendance in a period. A study of the psychometric properties of the Form-90 (Tonigan et al., 1997) found that this AA percentage measure had excellent test–retest consistency (Intraclass correlation coefficient = 0.62; $r = 0.92$) across a 2-day interval.

Consistency in self-report is critical, but it does not imply truthfulness. To examine the validity of self-reported AA attendance, information provided by two independent sources was compared. A condition of participation in Project MATCH was that clients provided the name of a collateral who could be interviewed periodically during the trial to corroborate client self-reports. One component of the collateral version of the

Form-90 interview focused on the collateral's estimation of the frequency of the client's AA meeting attendance. At intake, client and collateral estimates of the *exact* percentage of days of (client) AA attendance demonstrated significant but modest correspondence ($r = 0.62$, $n = 734$, Outpatient; $r = 0.35$, $n = 580$, Aftercare). Substantial improvement in client–collateral agreement, however, was found at subsequent assessments. Three months after treatment, for example, the correlation between clients and collaterals on AA attendance for the Outpatient and Aftercare arms had increased to 0.84 and 0.67, respectively. A similar pattern of convergence between client and collateral data has been reported for drinking outcomes as well (e.g., Miller et al., 1979), and may reflect enhanced vigilance among collaterals. Another explanation for improvements in client–collateral estimate is the common effect of treatment. Clients report increased abstinence after treatment and, jointly, collaterals expect that clients receiving treatment *should* be abstinent.

The unobserved nature of AA attendance may, in part, explain differences in client and collateral reports. To test this possibility, difference scores were computed by subtracting collateral reports of the frequency of client AA attendance from client self-reports of AA attendance (for intake, 3-month and six-month follow-ups). Positive mean difference scores could suggest that, on average, clients reported attending more AA meetings than collaterals were aware of, although client fabrication could also explain such a discrepancy. Nearly all difference scores were positive and modest in size. Combining these findings with the test–retest reliability data, it can be concluded that highly reliable and reasonably valid reports of AA meeting attendance were obtained in Project MATCH.

Alcoholics Anonymous Involvement Inventory (AAI)

Measures of AA attendance are likely to overestimate AA involvement because more people attend than actually become engaged and committed to Twelve Step principles and practices. Recognition of this bias has led to the development of instruments to directly assess involvement in AA (e.g., Morgenstern et al., 1996; Kingree, 1997; Humphreys et al., 1998). The AAI was developed in the planning stage of Project MATCH to measure the extent of past and current involvement in AA (Tonigan et al., 1996a). The AAI was administered at intake and at the 3-month, 9-month, and 15-month follow-ups. The self-report questionnaire is comprised of 13 items that inquire about meeting attendance, working the Twelve Steps, sponsorship, celebration of AA birthdays, and spiritual awakening. Test–retest findings suggest that clients consistently report specific AA activities that are distinct from attendance at meetings ($r = 0.98$). Examination of the baseline characteristics of the Project MATCH samples indicated that whereas lifetime (78%) and recent (50%) AA meeting attendance was relatively common before recruitment into the study, actual practice of the AA program (e.g., working the steps) was relatively uncommon (69% of the sample reported fewer than two AA steps completed in their lifetime).

Subjective ratings of Alcoholics Anonymous

Some people who attend AA do not become involved in the AA program and fellowship. Of those who do become involved, not all will feel that their AA participation is beneficial. Two measures were used to assess subjective ratings of the importance of AA attendance for achieving and maintaining sobriety. One item, administered immediately after treatment as part of a larger questionnaire, asked: '. . . how helpful was . . . encouragement to get involved in AA?' A second item, administered at the 3-month, 9-month, and 15-month follow-up interviews, asked clients to rate the importance of self-help group attendance for maintaining sobriety. Clients were asked this question only if they had a period of continuous abstinence of at least 14 days during the previous 3 months. Bivariate correlations among the three follow-up measures of 'usefulness of self-help groups such as AA' exhibited a wide range of agreement within clients across time ($r = 0.28$ to $r = 0.61$). Bivariate correlations between these usefulness measures and percentage of days AA meetings were attended, on the other hand, were strongly positive and significant, supporting convergent validity. It appears that subjective rating of the benefit of AA attendance varies as a function of time following formal treatment.

Results

Outpatient and Aftercare differences

A majority of the Project MATCH sample had prior AA exposure. Fifty percent of the clients reported attending at least one AA meeting in the year before study participation, and an additional 28% had gone to AA sometime earlier. Prior engagement in AA-related activities, however, was low: 69% of the sample had completed fewer than two of the Twelve Steps

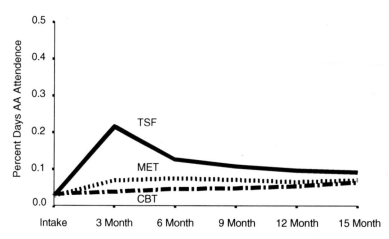

Figure 11.1 Percentage of days of Alcoholics Anonymous (AA) attendance during each 3-month follow-up period among Outpatient clients assigned to Cognitive–Behavioral Therapy (CBT), Motivation Enhancement Therapy (MET) and Twelve Step Facilitation therapy (TSF).

of AA, and only 10% reported completing four or more. Meeting attendance was low immediately before study recruitment. In the Aftercare sample, 71.6% of the clients reported no AA meeting attendance during the 90 days before study recruitment, a percentage that excluded consideration of possible AA attendance during their inpatient stay. Of the clients who did attend, the average number of AA meetings was 4.0. In the Outpatient sample, 75.1% of the clients reported no AA attendance during the 90 days before study recruitment, a percentage that took into consideration possible AA attendance before their most recent drink. Clients who did attend AA did so, on average, 2.66 days.

The percentage of days of AA meeting attendance for the three treatment conditions for the Outpatient and Aftercare samples are displayed in Figures 11.1 and 11.2, respectively. Seventy-five percent of the sample (Aftercare and Outpatient combined) reported attending AA at least once during the 12 months of post-treatment follow-up, and 23% of the sample reported AA attendance at all of the post-treatment interviews. At each assessment point, the Aftercare sample reported approximately twice as much AA attendance ($p < 0.05$) as the Outpatient sample. The higher rates of AA attendance among Aftercare clients may be due to the inpatient treatment experience, which generally encouraged clients to attend AA. Another possible reason is that Aftercare clients had completed inpatient

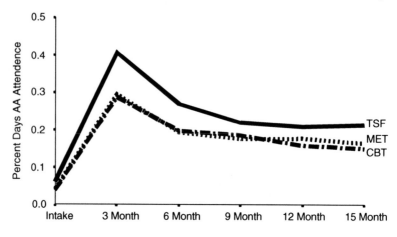

Figure 11.2 Percentage of days of Alcoholics Anonymous (AA) attendance during each 3-month follow-up period among Aftercare clients assigned to Cognitive–Behavioral Therapy (CBT), Motivational Enhancement Therapy (MET) and Twelve Step Facilitation therapy (TSF).

treatment. As a self-selected and highly motivated group of clients, they may have been more likely to seek the social support for abstinence offered by AA. Another explanation for the higher AA attendance among the Aftercare clients is suggested by findings in the AA affiliation literature (Humphreys et al., 1991; Emrick et al., 1993; Tonigan et al., 1996b; Morgenstern et al., 1996), which suggests that greater severity of alcohol dependence and alcohol-related problems is strongly predictive of Twelve Step participation. In Project MATCH, nearly all comparisons of the baseline characteristics of the Aftercare and Outpatient samples indicated that the Aftercare sample was more alcohol dependent and was more affected by the consequences of heavy alcohol consumption.

Treatment group differences

A central objective of TSF was to engage clients in AA. Clients assigned to CBT and MET, however, often elected to attend AA in addition to their formal treatment, and therapists in these conditions neither encouraged nor discouraged AA participation. Repeated measures analyses of variance (multivariate approach) were conducted to evaluate the relationship between AA meeting attendance and treatment assignment in the Aftercare sample. The model included a single within-subject factor (six levels;

percent AA attendance at intake and five follow-up points) and two between-subject factors, treatment assignment (three levels), and a Clinical Research Unit (CRU, five levels). CRU was included to control for cross-site variation within study arm. Although this term was significant in selected analyses reported in this chapter, implications of cross-site variability transcend the focus of this chapter and are not discussed. Main and first-order interaction effects were tested within the context of the full model, which included the time by CRU by treatment assignment term. Tests of simple effects used ψ_i error term, and orthogonal polynomial contrasts were conducted when levels of a between-subject factor were nested in the within-subject factor.

About 90% ($n = 853$) of the Outpatient sample was included in analyses examining AA attendance rates by treatment condition across time. TSF Outpatient clients reported significantly higher rates of attendance over the entire follow-up interval ($F(2, 850) = 16.06, p < 0.0001$), but the magnitude of this difference varied significantly across the 12 months of follow-up (interaction of treatment by time) ($F = (10, 1692) = 19.22, p < 0.0001$). TSF clients attended AA on more days than CBT and MET clients both during treatment (3 month, $p < 0.00001$) and during the three 3-month periods after the end of treatment (months 4–12, $p < 0.0001$, $p < 0.001$, and $p < 0.009$, respectively). However, no significant difference was found in the percentage of days of AA attendance during the last 3 months of the follow-up period (months 13–15, $p < 0.186$). Figures 11.1 and 11.2 suggest quite different patterns of attendance within the Outpatient MET and CBT conditions relative to the Aftercare CBT and MET groups. Specifically, clients assigned to the Outpatient CBT group did not report an increase in days of AA attendance during treatment, nor did they report a decay in attendance during the follow-up phase of the study. On the other hand, MET clients reported an increase during treatment in days of AA attendance (like their Aftercare counterparts), but attendance rates did not decay during follow-up in the Outpatient MET condition as they had in the Aftercare MET condition. It should be noted, however, that AA attendance remained higher (in all three treatment groups) in the Aftercare than in the Outpatient sample at 15 months.

Ninety percent ($n = 698$) of the Aftercare sample was followed up and had complete AA attendance data for the 15-month period. Collapsing across time periods, clients assigned to TSF reported significantly more days of AA attendance than the MET and CBT clients, ($F(2, 680) = 5.29$, $p < 0.005$). However, the magnitude of this treatment difference changed

Table 11.1. *Alcoholics Anonymous Involvement[a] by study arm and treatment condition at intake and at the 3-month, 9-month, and 15-month follow-up evaluations*

	Intake	3-month	9-month	15-month
Outpatient sample				
CBT	0.96	1.42	1.51	1.61
MET	0.94	1.57	1.83	1.91
TSF	0.95	2.92	2.48	2.40
Aftercare sample				
CBT	1.26	2.65	2.56	2.47
MET	1.37	2.69	2.59	2.50
TSF	1.34	3.50	3.26	3.08

[a]AA involvement is measured by the Alcoholics Anonymous Involvement scale (Tonigan et al., 1996a).
CBT, Cognitive–Behavioral Therapy; MET, Motivational Enhancement Therapy; TSF, Twelve Step Facilitation.

over time, as evidenced by a significant treatment by time interaction (F $(10, 1352) = 2.08$, $p < 0.023$). Clients in the three treatment conditions had significantly different AA attendance rates during treatment ($p < 0.004$, 3-month), and for the 3 months after treatment ($p < 0.007$, 6-month). As illustrated in Figure 11.2, TSF clients reported significantly more days of AA meeting attendance than either the MET or CBT clients. No differences in AA attendance were found between the three treatment groups at months 7–12, but TSF clients had significantly more AA attendance during the last 3 months of follow-up ($p < 0.024$, months 13–15). A substantial increase in AA attendance during treatment was followed, in all conditions, by a marked decay in attendance in the first 3 months after treatment. The location in time of a second decline in AA attendance varied by treatment condition over the 12 months of follow-up.

Table 11.1 shows the baseline and follow-up mean values by arm and treatment group for the composite AAI measure. The composite score aggregates responses to 13 items inquiring about specific AA activities (e.g., having or being a sponsor, attending '90 meetings in 90 days,' celebrating an AA sobriety birthday, completing the Twelve Steps). The composite score ranges from 0 to 13. The means presented in the table are for those cases with complete data across all assessment points (Outpatient = 47%, Aftercare = 62%). Mean differences between cases with complete data at all time points and cases with complete data at selected points were slight and without apparent upward or downward bias ($p > 0.05$).

Analyses of variance (multivariate approach) were conducted to examine the between-group pattern of mean AAI scores across the follow-up period. The design included a single within-subject factor (four levels; composite AAI involvement at intake, 3-month, 9-month, and 15-month follow-up points) and two between-subject factors, treatment assignment (three levels) and CRU (five levels). Collapsing across time in the Aftercare sample, TSF clients reported more involvement in AA activities than did clients assigned to the CBT and MET groups ($F(2, 461) = 7.42, p < 0.001$). The magnitude of this between-group difference, however, changed during the 15 months of the study (treatment by time interaction, Wilks (6, 918) = 3.47, $p < 0.002$). TSF clients consistently reported practicing AA activities more often than CBT and MET clients at three assessment points: months 3 ($p < 0.0001$), 9 ($p < 0.001$), and 15 ($p < 0.011$). However, the difference declined in magnitude over time. As indicated in Table 11.1, a sharp increase in AA involvement in each of the therapies during treatment was followed by a decline across the 12 months of follow-up.

Analysis of AA involvement by treatment condition in the Outpatient sample was based upon those clients providing complete AAI data at intake and at the 3-month, 9-month, and 15-month follow-ups (47%, $n = 446$). Clients assigned to the TSF condition reported practicing AA-related activities significantly more than CBT and MET clients over the entire 15-month period ($F(2, 431) = 23.45, p < 0.0001$). A significant group by time interaction (Wilks (6, 856) = 18.45, $p < 0.001$), however, indicated that this difference was moderated across follow-up assessment points. Clients assigned to TSF reported significantly more AA-related activities during the 12 weeks of treatment ($p < 0.0001$), and for the 12 months after treatment (months 4–6, $p < 0.0001$; months 7–9, $p < 0.001$; months 13–15, $p < 0.001$). As with the Aftercare clients, there was a sharp increase in AA-related activities for all clients during treatment, followed by a decay in mean AAI scores.

Evaluation of treatment

All clients were asked to complete an evaluation of their treatment at 3-month follow-up. One item asked respondents to rate on a five-point scale (ranging from 'extremely helpful' to 'extremely unhelpful') the encouragement they received to attend AA. Because such encouragement was not included in the CBT and MET protocols, clients were offered a 'not applicable' option. Not surprisingly, in the Outpatient sample, 43% of the CBT and 36% of the MET clients responded that the item was not applicable to their Project MATCH experience. In the Aftercare sample, however, only 14% of CBT clients and 8% of MET clients chose the 'not applicable' option, suggesting that clients were considering both prior inpatient treatment and Project MATCH participation when responding.

Seventy-six percent ($n = 591$) of the Aftercare sample was included in a one-way ANOVA with ratings of 'helpfulness' of AA encouragement as the dependent measure and treatment group as the between-subject factor. The omnibus test was significant ($p < 0.001$), and follow-up tests indicated that TSF clients rated AA encouragement as significantly more helpful than did either MET or CBT clients. On average, TSF clients rated 'Encouragement to attend AA' as 'moderately helpful,' with MET and CBT clients reporting that such encouragement was between neutral and moderately helpful in attaining treatment goals. The findings were identical using the same analytical approach in the Outpatient sample ($n = 644$, 68%).

Patterns of Alcoholics Anonymous utilization

The findings presented thus far have been based on treatment group comparisons. In this section, we address patterns of AA utilization. Regardless of treatment assignment, clients had the option not to attend AA at all or, alternatively, could participate in AA activities as much or as little as they chose. The following six categories were created to represent AA participation within the Project MATCH experience:

1. no AA attendance (months 1–15);
2. AA attendance during treatment (months 1–3), no AA after treatment (months 4–15);
3. AA attendance during treatment and follow-up, but AA disaffiliation occurring by the end of the ninth month of follow-up (month 12);
4. AA attendance during treatment and all follow-ups (months 1–15);
5. no AA attendance during treatment, but some AA attendance during follow-up (months 4–15);
6. other (i.e., a pattern, usually erratic, that did not fit the first five categories).

Table 11.2. *Classification of Project MATCH clients according to Alcoholics Anonymous (AA) participation*[a]

	No AA (%) 1–15	AA (%) 1–3	AA (%) 1–12	AA (%) 1–15	AA (%) 4–15	Other (%)
Aftercare sample						
CBT ($n = 242$)	15	14	15	36	1	19
MET ($n = 232$)	13	13	16	36	2	21
TSF ($n = 224$)	5	14	14	46	1	20
Outpatient sample						
CBT ($n = 274$)	55	4	5	8	7	21
MET ($n = 274$)	52	4	9	9	8	18
TSF ($n = 305$)	19	24	17	26	0	15

[a]The column headings represent five different types of AA participation during the Project MATCH study. These groups were as follows: (1) no AA attendance (months 1–15), (2) AA attendance during treatment (months 1–3), no AA attendance after treatment (months 4–15), (3) AA attendance during treatment and follow-up (months 4–12), (4) AA attendance during treatment and all follow-up months, and (5) other. The percentages in parentheses indicate the proportion of clients assigned to a treatment condition who belong to a given AA utilization group. The column headed 'Other' identifies the percentages of cases that could not be classified into the previous categories. These cases did report AA attendance during at least 1 month of the 15 months of the Project MATCH study, but such attendance was erratically spaced with months of non-AA attendance.
CBT, Cognitive–Behavioral Therapy; MET, Motivational Enhancement Therapy; TSF, Twelve Step Facilitation.

Table 11.2 presents the results according to study arm and treatment condition. Approximately 10% of the cases ($n = 177$) were excluded from the analysis because complete AA attendance data at each assessment point were unavailable to classify clients according to the nature of their AA participation. The column heading 'Other' shows the percentage of cases that did not fit into the first five categories. These cases did report AA attendance during at least one of the 15 months of the study, but such attendance was erratically spaced with months of non-AA attendance.

The table shows that for all three treatment conditions and both study arms, relatively few clients initiated AA attendance *after* the 12 weeks of treatment. The figures clearly demonstrate that if participation in AA is not initiated during treatment, only a handful of clients (see column labeled AA months 4–15) subsequently initiate AA attendance after treatment. In the Outpatient TSF condition, however, the data indicate that AA attendance during treatment in and of itself does not guarantee sustained AA participation. In this regard, 41% of the Outpatient TSF clients who did initiate AA attendance during treatment (AA months 1–3) discontinued their AA attendance either at the end of treatment (24%, AA months 1–3) or during the first 9 months after treatment (17%, AA months 1–12). As noted above, Aftercare clients attended AA significantly more often than Outpatient clients.

The patterns of AA utilization observed in these data raise additional questions about AA attendance and involvement: was there a threshold in the frequency of AA attendance during treatment that would predict sustained participation, and how was sustained AA participation manifested in meeting attendance and other AA activities?

In the Aftercare sample, a clear linear trend was found between AA attendance during and after treatment. Clients attending AA meetings on 6 or fewer days (of 90) during treatment tended to discontinue meeting attendance after treatment. Clients reporting AA meeting attendance for about 28% (25 days) of the 90 days of treatment continued attendance at AA meetings into the post-treatment phase of the study, but discontinued AA attendance within 9 months. It is noteworthy that median AA attendance for this group declined rapidly across the follow-up assessment intervals. Finally, clients reporting AA meeting attendance for all of the 12 follow-up months also reported having attended AA meetings nearly 50% (45 days) of the available days during the 12 weeks of treatment. Nevertheless, clients demonstrating sustained AA attendance throughout follow-up also reduced their AA attendance over time.

The AAI measure also showed that increased participation in the Twelve Step program activities during treatment predicted post-treatment engagement in AA. In addition, there was a different pattern of AAI median scores within each AA utilization group across time, and these patterns were related to AA attendance. Median AAI scores declined steadily across time in those AA classification groups that attended AA during treatment but discontinued AA meeting attendance after treatment (AA months 1–3, AA months 1–12). In contrast, practice of AA activities increased for those clients who sustained AA meeting attendance throughout the 12-month follow-up *despite* somewhat reduced AA meeting attendance.

Like the Aftercare sample, median days of AA attendance during treatment was a strong predictor of post-treatment AA attendance in the Outpatient sample as well. Clients who attended AA only during treatment went to AA on less than 10% of the available days of the 12 weeks of treatment. Clients who continued their AA attendance into follow-up, but not for the entire 12-month period, typically went to AA on 18% of the available days during treatment. Outpatient clients with sustained AA attendance throughout the follow-up period typically attended AA on 35% of the available days during treatment. As in the Aftercare sample, AA attendance by Outpatient clients declined across the 12-month follow-up period, even for those reporting sustained AA attendance. Like the Aftercare sample, disaffiliation with AA was associated with declining involvement in or practicing of AA-related activities. Clients reporting sustained AA attendance, however, reported significant increases in AA-related activities *despite* reductions in the frequency of AA meeting attendance.

Alcoholics Anonymous attendance and alcohol use

The relationship between AA attendance and abstinence has been the subject of some debate. On the one hand, it has been argued that AA is the most effective method to manage recovery from alcoholism (e.g., Snyder, 1980; Hudson, 1985). On the other hand, it has been argued that AA is helpful to only 5% of the people who choose to affiliate with the organization (Bufe, 1991). Most alcoholism treatment programs in the USA refer their clients to AA, and the legal system has increasingly used it as a resource, despite claims that this interferes with the separation of church and state. Indeed, strong opinions – pro and con – are the rule rather than the exception when discussing the utility of AA affiliation and involvement. Reviewing 31 studies examining AA attendance after treatment, Emrick and colleagues (1993) concluded that AA attendance and abstinence were modestly and positively related ($r = 0.21$). Tonigan et al. (1996b) re-examined these 31 studies, dividing them according to whether the sample was drawn from an inpatient or an outpatient setting. AA attendance was more strongly associated with abstinence after inpatient treatment ($r = 0.21$) than after outpatient treatment ($r = 0.15$). Two-thirds of the AA studies ($n = 0.20$), however, were judged to be of poor methodologic quality, which was attributed to an over-reliance on samples of convenience, the use of unvalidated assessment tools, and the failure to corroborate self-report information about drinking and AA attendance.

In contrast, substantial confidence can be placed in the findings of Project MATCH relating to AA. Measures of AA attendance and involvement were subjected to rigorous reliability and validity checks. In 48% of prior published reports (Emrick et al., 1993), there was no evaluation at all of the consistency and accuracy of self-reported AA affiliation and involvement. Substantial effort was also expended in Project MATCH to determine the reliability and validity of self-reported alcohol consumption during and after treatment (Tonigan et al., 1997; Babor et al., 2000).

It is encouraging that global estimates of the association between AA attendance and alcohol use in Project MATCH compare favorably in direction and magnitude with prior meta-analytic reviews. In particular, frequency of AA attendance (months 1–3 and 4–6) and Percent Days Abstinent (PDA; months 1–6) were positively related in both the Outpatient ($r = 0.22$ at 3 months; $r = 0.23$ at 6 months) and Aftercare samples ($r = 0.20$ at 3 months; $r = 0.28$ at 6 months). Frequency of AA attendance was also associated with a higher number of abstinent days during the later (distal) follow-up period (months 7–15). Estimates of association for this time period ranged from $r = 0.19$ (months 10–12) to $r = 0.24$ (months 13–15) for the Outpatient sample and from $r = 0.31$ (months 10–12) to $r = 0.26$ (months 13–15) for the Aftercare sample. Measures of drinking intensity (Drinks per Drinking Day, DDD) provide a similar picture. AA attendance is associated with significantly less drinking when drinking occurs, whether at proximal or distal follow-up periods.

Earlier meta-analytic reviewers had speculated that the benefits of AA may be moderated by the type of formal treatment clients receive, based on the rationale that formal treatment in a Twelve Step program would be associated with stronger relationships between AA attendance and abstinence. Conversely, formal treatment not incorporating a Twelve Step orientation should reduce the association between AA attendance and abstinence. A series of hierarchical multiple regression analyses (MRA) was conducted to test this hypothesis. Four MRAs were conducted within each study arm. Two primary dependent measures, PDA and DDD, were used to represent proximal (months 1–6) and distal (months 7–12) drinking status. Each of the four dependent measures was separately and sequentially regressed on six sets of variables within each MRA. Categorical independent variables were effect coded, and construction of product terms followed recommendations made by Pedhuaser (1982). The order of independent variables was: (1) CRU or site effect, (2) treatment main effect, (3) site by treatment effect, (4) baseline measures of both PDA and

DDD, (5) two measures of percent days AA attendance, one for each of the two 3-month increments included in proximal or distal follow-up, and (6) the interaction terms for AA attendance by treatment main effect.

In the Aftercare sample, the analyses did not support the hypothesis. Positive associations between AA attendance and abstinence, and negative associations between AA attendance and drinking intensity, were found in all three Project MATCH treatments. But differences in the magnitudes of these associations were not sufficient to exceed chance fluctuation.

A slightly different picture emerged in the Outpatient sample. AA attendance was positively associated with abstinence (PDA) regardless of the Project MATCH treatment received. A differential benefit consistent with the hypothesis was found, however, between AA attendance and drinking intensity (DDD) by treatment condition. Specifically, there was a strong negative association between AA attendance and number of drinks consumed when drinking occurred among TSF clients at both the proximal (months 1–6) and distal (months 7–12) follow-ups. To a lesser degree, this relationship was also found among MET clients. In contrast, CBT clients reported a positive relationship between drinking intensity and AA attendance during proximal follow-up (i.e., those attending more AA meetings were actually drinking more). This relationship did not persist into distal follow-up. Interpretation of this finding is difficult because the data do not permit ascertainment of the temporal order between drinking and AA attendance. Although conflicting ideologies may have resulted in more drinking, it is equally plausible that clients who were faring poorly (drinking heavily) in CBT elected to attend AA as another attempt to alter their drinking.

AA is an abstinence-based, mutual-help program. Did AA meeting attendance predict complete abstinence? Five logistic regressions were conducted separately for the Outpatient and Aftercare samples. The criterion measure, abstinence (yes/no), was computed by recoding the Composite outcome measure (Zweben & Cisler, 1996; Project MATCH Research Group, 1997a) into a two-level categorical variable (total abstinence versus drinking of any kind, which included non-problematic and problematic alcohol consumption). CRU and treatment group assignment were effect coded and entered into the regression model prior to the AA attendance term (percent days AA meeting attendance).

In the Aftercare sample, frequency of AA meeting attendance was positively and significantly predictive of total abstinence during treatment ($p < 0.0001$) and at all follow-up points ($p < 0.001$ in all cases). Similarly, in the Outpatient sample, total abstinence during treatment ($p < 0.01$) and at all follow-up periods ($p < 0.001$) was significantly and positively related to frequency of AA meeting attendance.

Discussion

This chapter describes the AA experience of Project MATCH clients. The findings provide compelling evidence for the value of AA as an adjunct to professional treatment, and suggest practical ways to maximize the potential benefits of AA through TSF. Seventy-five percent of the Project MATCH sample reported at least some AA exposure after study recruitment, and 23% reported attending AA continuously during the 12 months of follow-up. It is noteworthy that the therapeutic modality with the lowest rate of AA attendance, Outpatient CBT, still had a substantial proportion of clients (45%) reporting some AA attendance either during or after treatment. Clearly, a majority of clients in this multisite study regarded AA as a valuable resource.

The findings presented in this chapter suggest that AA engagement is best considered a latent construct consisting of multiple dimensions, two of which are the frequency of attendance and the practice of AA-related activities. The TSF treatment was quite effective in increasing client behavior within each of these dimensions. Large differences in AA attendance rates were observed among TSF, CBT, and MET during the 12 weeks of treatment in both the Aftercare and Outpatient samples, and Outpatient TSF clients reported significantly higher rates of attendance than did MET or CBT clients throughout the 12-month follow-up period. Treatment group differences in AA attendance diminished in the Aftercare sample during the same period. It is noteworthy, however, that the measure of Aftercare involvement (rather than mere attendance) continued to differentiate TSF from MET and CBT clients throughout the 12 months of follow-up in both arms of the trial. Thus, whereas the differential effect of TSF therapy on AA attendance was not sustained in the Aftercare sample, TSF therapy was more effective in maintaining involvement in AA activities among both Outpatient and Aftercare clients. This is a further indication that AA involvement may be a more sensitive measure than attendance *per se* (cf. Montgomery et al., 1995).

One way to explain the steady decline in mean AA attendance rates across follow-ups is disaffiliation from AA. A substantial drop-out from AA did occur at the end of formal treatment. This attrition was most pronounced in the Outpatient TSF condition, where 24% of the clients who had attended AA during treatment reported no further AA attendance during the 12 months of follow-up. No other 3-month interval during follow-up had as high an AA disaffiliation rate. Nevertheless, the absolute number of persons attending AA remained relatively stable after the midpoint of the follow-up phase of the study. The clear implication is that the same number of clients were attending AA (i.e., had not disaffiliated), but they were attending AA less often. For clients who continued to attend at least some AA meetings during each follow-up period, AA involvement actually increased while mean AA meeting attendance declined. It appears that the relative importance of frequent meeting attendance gave way to greater engagement in AA-related activities and principles. Newcomers to AA are typically advised to attend 90 meetings in 90 days. After this initiation phase, however, meeting attendance diminishes considerably, and is expected to do so. The 1996 national survey of AA members found that the average number of AA meetings attended is fewer than three meetings per week (Alcoholics Anonymous, 1997).

Yet AA attendance *per se* is far from irrelevant. The AA utilization profiles derived from the Project MATCH data showed that if post-treatment AA attendance is desired, it is vital that clients initiate AA attendance during treatment. Only a handful of Aftercare and Outpatient clients initiated AA attendance after the end of formal treatment. Furthermore, infrequent AA attendance during treatment does not appear to be sufficient for engagement. The findings suggest that continued AA attendance during follow-up is most likely to occur when meetings are attended on more than one-third of the available days in treatment (i.e., more than 2 days per week). Another clinically relevant observation is that the risk for AA disaffiliation is greatest at the point when clients are exiting treatment. This was especially the case for Outpatient TSF clients. The findings suggest that if therapists want their clients to be involved in AA after treatment, they should see that AA attendance begins during treatment, and encourage clients to attend three or more meetings per week during treatment. Some brief follow-up checks may also be warranted within the first months after treatment to minimize attrition. This kind of simple initiative may substantially increase the likelihood that clients will attend meetings and continue with AA (e.g., Sisson & Mallams, 1981).

What can be said of the benefits associated with AA attendance? Global bivariate correlations confirm some of the major conclusions of earlier meta-analytic work (Emrick et al., 1993; Tonigan et al., 1996b). In the case of Project MATCH, corroborated measures of AA attendance and drinking outcome indicate that small-to-modest benefits were associated with frequency of AA attendance after formal treatment. AA attendance was significantly associated with abstinent days and reduced DDD. We note that the 'benefits' identified here pertain only to abstinence, which is considered in AA to be a necessary prerequisite but in some ways only a small part of sobriety. Research is needed to understand the relationships among AA involvement, abstinence, and the kind of sobriety more broadly conceived by AA.

With one notable exception, the relative benefit associated with AA affiliation did not vary in relation to the kind of treatment clients received. This finding was consistent for both Aftercare and Outpatient clients. It is not clear why Outpatient CBT clients reported an adverse association between frequency of AA attendance and intensity of drinking at proximal follow-up. A similar finding has been noted by other researchers in somewhat different contexts (Humphreys et al., 1999) and certainly warrants further attention.

In conclusion, clients participating in Project MATCH regarded AA as an important community-based resource. Analyses of AA participation and involvement indicated that TSF increased the frequency of AA attendance and the practice of AA-related activities. Despite the decline in AA attendance after the formal treatment period, TSF continued to sustain involvement and commitment to AA. The findings suggest that one reason TSF seems to be effective is because it encourages and initiates AA affiliation during a critical period of receptivity to constructive action. If such action is not taken during this critical period, meaningful AA affiliation is unlikely to occur afterwards.

Part III
Conclusions and Implications

12

Summary and conclusions

WILLIAM R. MILLER AND RICHARD LONGABAUGH

This chapter summarizes the findings of Project MATCH, concluding that they are both encouraging and humbling. Three very different treatment methods were associated with similarly positive outcomes. Client traits did not prove to be significant prognostic factors; instead, malleable states such as motivation and social support were the most predictive. Alcoholics Anonymous involvement was associated with better outcomes. Support was modest for the popular idea of matching clients to optimal treatments on the basis of their pretreatment characteristics. Twelve Step Facilitation (TSF) was more effective than one or both of the other treatments with: (a) Outpatient clients without additional psychopathology, (b) Outpatients with high social support for continued drinking, and (c) Aftercare clients high in alcohol dependence. Motivational Enhancement Therapy was more effective than the other treatments for Outpatients high in anger. Cognitive–Behavioral Therapy was more effective than TSF for Aftercare clients low in alcohol dependence. For those who devote their lives to helping others recover from alcohol abuse and dependence, many perplexing questions remain.

It is challenging in a book, let alone in one chapter, to summarize what is important from a study the size of Project MATCH. The largest controlled trial of psychotherapies ever conducted, it involved 261 staff working over a period of 10 years with 1726 clients of outpatient and residential treatment facilities at nine sites. During this time, the project has generated more than 125 published articles, chapters, and monographs.

In this chapter we bring together the findings of Project MATCH regarding: (1) trial integrity, (2) overall client outcomes, (3) main effects, (4) matching effects, (5) therapist effects, (6) prognostic client characteristics, (7) Alcoholics Anonymous (AA) involvement, and (8) variability across sites. Finally, we draw some broad conclusions from the trial, which is expanded upon in the final chapter of this volume.

How credible was the trial?

Given the significant investment of public funds required to carry out a national study of this scope, great care was taken to protect both the integrity (internal validity) and generalizability (external validity) of the trial. A large sample was recruited, representing a broad range of clients seeking help for alcohol problems. The 80 therapists likewise represented a diversity of backgrounds, with education ranging from PhD psychologists to recovering counselors without college degrees.

Measures for the trial were carefully chosen. Most had been used in many previous studies and had well-documented psychometric properties. For key dependent variables, we designed new instruments combining what had been learned from prior research. For these we conducted a special sub-study (Del Boca & Brown, 1996) demonstrating high test–retest reliability and internal consistency for measures of drinking, drug use, consequences, dependence, motivation, religiosity, and AA involvement. Similarly encouraging were our findings regarding the convergence of different measures for the same constructs. A particular focus here was verification of the accuracy of client self-reports, through collateral interviews with significant others and through analysis of breath and blood samples. These analyses (Babor et al., 2000) strongly supported the validity of what Project MATCH clients told us about their outcomes.

Another strength of the trial was a high rate of retention in assessment. We were able to determine outcomes for over 90% of all clients who had been entered into the trial, at follow-up points at 3, 6, 9, 12, and 15 months. In fact, 89.9% of clients provided data for all five points (Babor et al., 2000). At a longer follow-up with outpatients at 39 months, outcomes were once again ascertained for over 90% of the sample. High completion rates were also achieved for blood samples and collateral interviews, yielding credibility that reported findings do accurately represent outcomes of the full Project MATCH population.

It is important in any trial to know what treatments were actually delivered. Great care was taken to ensure that the three treatments tested in this study were conducted in a consistent and replicable manner. Detailed therapist manuals were prepared and published for all three treatments (Kadden et al., 1992a; Miller et al., 1992; Nowinski et al., 1992). All sessions were routinely videotaped and were supervised at both the local and the national level. Central clinical supervisors, who monitored therapist performance at all sites throughout the trial, had and used the authority to withdraw therapists from the trial if adherence to treatment protocols fell below standards. Coding of videotapes by independent observers, who were unaware of treatment assignment, showed clear discriminability of the treatments, documenting many differences among the therapies that were consistent with the theory and practice of the three manualized therapies. Clients seemed to appreciate all three treatments equally, giving similar satisfaction ratings across conditions. This satisfaction was also reflected in uniformly high rates of retention in treatment, with clients completing, on average, two-thirds of all planned sessions.

To what extent did Project MATCH clients resemble those treated in routine clinical settings across the USA? A few specific subpopulations seen in clinical settings were not included in the Project MATCH sample. Most notably, clients who had other concurrent substance-dependence diagnoses were excluded, although clients with drug-abuse diagnoses were included. Also, clients with currently acute psychosis were excluded from the project, and so Project MATCH findings may not generalize to this particular group. Yet a broad range of concomitant psychopathology was represented in the sample, and 'dual diagnosis' was the norm. In severity of alcohol-use disorders, Project MATCH clients covered a wide range, likely to encompass the presenting characteristics of clients at most private and public outpatient and residential treatment programs. Given the broad range of clients, the mean values may not resemble those of programs that serve a more selected clientele, but proxies for most treatment populations can be found within the trial's diversity. Heterogeneity of clients was sought specifically to enhance the ability to detect client–treatment matches.

There is also more direct evidence of the representativeness of the sample. At several sites, clients enrolling in Project MATCH were compared with those served at the same clinical facility but not enrolled in the trial. Differences in characteristics were generally small, and not consistent across sites. At one site, clients from the same facility who were enrolled in the trial were compared to those not enrolled on baseline attributes as well as aggregate outcomes. Few differences were observed (Velasquez et al., 2000). Finally, the attributes and outcomes of Project MATCH clients were compared with those for other large clinical trials from the alcoholism field, again suggesting that there is nothing unrepresentative or highly selective in the present study. There is every reason to believe that clients treated in Project MATCH are generally representative of those treated in US outpatient and residential facilities.

What happened to clients after treatment?

As one examines the outcome graphs from Project MATCH (Chapters 7 and 8), the most obvious differences are those changes shown by clients in all three treatment conditions between baseline and the end of treatment at 3-month follow-up. Overall drinking plummets. There was a fourfold increase in abstinent days from six to about 24 per month. Before treatment, clients averaged about 15 drinks on days when they drank, and showed a fivefold decrease to average about three Drinks per Drinking Day (DDD) after treatment. Over follow-up intervals as long as 3 years, maintenance of these changes was excellent. At 39 months, Outpatients were still collectively averaging 69% abstinent days.

At 15 months, the longest follow-up for the entire sample, 30.4% of Outpatients and 45.9% of Aftercare clients had been abstaining completely for 3 months or more. Another 12.4% of Outpatients and 7.3% of Aftercare clients were drinking moderately and without problems. Continuous abstinence (no drinking at all since the end of treatment) was reported by 13.8% of Outpatients and 26.7% of Aftercare clients at 15 months. For Outpatients at 39 months, 29.4% reported complete abstinence during the previous 3 months.

The breadth of outcome measures confirmed that this improvement was not restricted to alcohol use. Clients also showed significant decreases in the use of illicit drugs, in depression and in alcohol-related problems, as well as improvement in liver function and in psychosocial functioning (see Chapter 9).

Could the outcomes of Project MATCH clients be characterized as atypical? There is no reason to believe so. Several other multisite studies have documented the outcomes of alcoholism treatment during the past four decades. All show that while complete abstinence is the exception rather than the rule, treated clients as a group do mostly abstain, drinking far less often, and when they do, usually drinking less and for shorter spans of time (Miller et al., 2001). They echo the Project MATCH finding that, at any given follow-up point, about a third to a half of clients are unambiguously in remission (abstaining, or drinking moderately and/or without problems). The pattern of generalized improvement following alcohol-focused treatment has also been widely replicated. The outcomes observed in Project MATCH do not appear to be substantially different from those in other well-documented treatment studies.

Did the treatments differ in outcome?

At the onset of the trial, only one of the three treatments, Cognitive–Behavioral Therapy (CBT), had clear empirical support for its general effectiveness (Miller et al., 1995a). Although the efficacy of brief interventions, such as Motivational Enhancement Therapy (MET), had been strongly supported for clients with less severe alcohol problems (Bien et al., 1993), its effectiveness with clients at more severe problem levels was not as well established. The Minnesota Model, from which the Twelve Step Facilitation (TSF) therapy was derived, had not been subjected to rigorous randomized clinical trials, despite favorable outcomes reported in naturalistic treatment studies (e.g., Hoffmann & Miller, 1992; Miller & Hoffmann, 1995). Thus, how TSF would fare relative to CBT or MET was unclear. Because of CBT's well-grounded empirical support, it was anticipated that any main effects of treatment that emerged were likely to favor CBT. Instead, we found that in both arms of the study the three treatments were not substantially different in their effectiveness. If any of the three treatments had a slight advantage, it was TSF, especially when compared on measures of outcome pertaining to continuous abstinence. MET yielded similar outcomes to those for CBT across the broad spectrum of the client population, both in the Aftercare and Outpatient settings. Given its relative brevity, this placed MET in a slightly more favorable position as a cost-effective treatment for a typical client (see Chapter 4).

When measures other than drinking were considered, the three treatments were also comparable in the outcomes they achieved. A conclusion to be drawn from these results is that any of the three individual therapies may suffice as a treatment for a broad spectrum of clients, at least if the treatments are delivered as they were in Project MATCH. However, a major question that remains is whether the intensive and frequent research assessments in all three treatments served as an active ingredient of treatment to dampen differences that might otherwise have emerged. This is clearly an important question for further research.

What client–treatment matches were found?

The primary aim of the study was to test whether client–treatment matching would improve clients' drinking outcomes. We therefore put a major effort into the development of *a priori* matching hypotheses that were based upon existing empirical research and sound theory. As described in

Chapter 6, the primary hypotheses selected by the Steering Committee included all those that had yielded promising matching results in prior studies of the treatments included in Project MATCH (Mattson et al., 1994). A set of secondary matching hypotheses was also developed and tested. Intensive effort was devoted to developing sound rationales for each of the hypotheses (Longabaugh & Wirtz, 2001). The rigorous research design and large sample maximized the likelihood of detecting any unambiguous matching effects (Donovan & Mattson, 1994).

Because of the rigor and scope of this effort, we were surprised to find support for only four matching effects. Three of these pertain to Outpatients. The most consistent matching effect was related to client anger: MET was more effective for clients with high anger than was CBT or TSF, but less effective for those with low anger. This is consistent with the expectation that the non-confrontational approach of MET would differentially benefit angry clients by diminishing their resistance.

A second observed matching effect is noteworthy in two respects. We found that TSF was more effective than MET for clients with networks supportive of their drinking, but not for those with networks already unsupportive of the clients' drinking. The first noteworthy aspect of this finding is that it did not emerge clearly until the third year after treatment. Had we ended our follow-ups at 1 year, this effect would never have been identified. Secondly, through causal chain analysis, we were able to establish that AA involvement was a significant factor underlying this matching effect. TSF was superior, in part, because of its greater success in getting clients with networks highly supportive of drinking involved in AA. For clients with networks unsupportive of drinking, AA involvement was not related to outcome.

The third matching effect of clinical significance is the superior effectiveness of TSF over CBT for Outpatient clients who do not have concomitant psychiatric impairment. At least during the first 9 months after treatment, clients low in Psychiatric Severity fared better in TSF than in CBT treatment.

Among Aftercare clients, only one substantial matching effect was observed, and it endured over the entire year of post-treatment follow-up. As hypothesized, CBT was more effective than TSF for clients with relatively low dependence symptoms, whereas TSF was more effective than CBT for clients having high dependence.

What is to be said about the lack of confirmation of so many other promising matching hypotheses? First, we did find some evidence of small matching effects for several of these, but such effects were not consistent over time. For example, one credible matching effect, for the variable Self-efficacy Confidence regarding abstinence, was present only during treatment: Outpatient clients low in Self-efficacy regarding abstinence fared better in TSF or CBT than in MET; nevertheless, once treatment was completed, the low Self-efficacy CBT and TSF clients resumed drinking at levels comparable to their counterparts treated in MET.

Other hypothesized matching effects were evident only for short periods of time, such as immediately after treatment (Sociopathy), during the middle of the follow-up period (e.g., Meaning Seeking), or at the end of the 1-year follow-up (e.g., Motivational Readiness to Change). Finally, some matching effects appeared in a direction opposite to that predicted; most notably, lower social functioning clients did best in TSF and poorest in CBT from the beginning of treatment through the entire year of follow-up. Other matching effects opposite to predictions occurred over shorter periods of time. For example, with clients lower in initial motivation, MET was less effective than CBT immediately following treatment. This pattern reversed to the predicted direction by the final months of follow-up.

Why did so many matching hypotheses fail to find support? Our causal chain analyses indicated that most often the breakdown was not a failure in theory *per se* (Finney, 1995), but occurred because the three treatments failed to differentially affect clients in the ways we had anticipated (Longabaugh & Wirtz, 2001). Short-term changes during treatment that were hypothesized to predict subsequent drinking outcomes often did so. It appears that either the active ingredients of the three treatments were less specific than we had thought, or that these active ingredients provided different pathways for particular kinds of clients to achieve similarly successful outcomes.

More generally, any of three explanations may account for why robust matching effects were not observed more often. First, features of the research design may have mitigated or masked matching effects that do occur in naturalistic settings. The intensity of research assessment is a consideration here. Second, it may simply be that matching clients on the basis of single client characteristics to one or another of the three individual therapies implemented in Project MATCH is not a fruitful approach to enhance outcomes. This explanation is strengthened by one of the few instances in which robust matching did occur. The superior effectiveness of TSF for clients with networks supportive of drinking was due, in part, to this treatment being more successful in getting clients involved in AA, an event that can be facilitated by treatment but which lies outside of the therapy itself (Longabaugh et al., 1998). It may be that matching predicated solely upon differential processes taking place in individual therapy (just one small event in the life of an alcoholic) is unlikely to affect client outcomes. A third possibility is that current theories of matching are insufficiently developed to specify the necessary set of circumstances under which matching will and will not occur. Certainly, the complexity of the matching results we did find, combined with our inability to fully account for this complexity, provides ample evidence of underspecification in current theory.

One comforting implication for current practice is that any of these three treatments, when implemented as they have been in Project MATCH, should be able to produce drinking outcomes comparable to those observed here, irrespective of single characteristics of the client. With a few exceptions noted above, mismatching to these three treatments does not appear to be a significant clinical problem.

Did therapists make a difference?

In all three of the treatments, in one arm of the trial or the other, and during or after treatment, clients' outcomes were significantly influenced by the therapist to whom they were assigned. Such difference in outcomes among therapists has been reported in several previous studies of substance abuse treatment (Najavits & Weiss, 1994). The surprise here was that in all but one of these analyses, the significant differences were accounted for by a single outlier therapist (not always the same person) whose outcomes differed from all the rest. Usually this was in the direction of the therapist's clients doing significantly worse than those of other therapists delivering the same treatment. This finding of negative outliers has also been reported elsewhere (e.g., McLellan et al., 1988).

Although some therapist traits were linked to outcomes within particular treatment modalities, there was no consistency across therapies. Our analyses detected no significant difference in outcomes for clients of therapists who were not themselves recovering alcoholics; that is, personal recovery status did not render an individual either a more or a less effective therapist. This is consistent with the findings of many other studies (McLellan et al., 1988).

Who did well?

Many of the client characteristics were selected for matching because they had shown prognostic significance in other studies. It could be expected that those that did not show matching effects would maintain their status as prognostic indicators. Whereas this expectation was largely borne out, some findings were surprising.

No single variable captured any sizable proportion of unique variance in predicting drinking outcomes. The strongest prognostic indicators were indices of motivational readiness, which uniquely accounted for no more than 3% of the variance in 3-year outcomes. The most consistent prognostic indicator was Self-Efficacy Temptation minus Confidence, which predicted both frequency and intensity of drinking at all follow-up intervals in both study arms.

Prognostic indicators in one arm of the study were generally not the same as those in the other arm. Only Self-efficacy Temptation minus Confidence and Support for Drinking were predictive of 1-year drinking outcomes in both arms of the study. Several variables had prognostic value in one arm of the study but not in the other. In the Outpatient arm, greater severity of alcohol problems predicted better long-term drinking outcomes at the 3-year follow-up. Alcohol Involvement and Alcohol Dependence were both predictive of a greater percentage of days abstinent, and Involvement was predictive of fewer drinks on a drinking day. Measures of Spirituality and Religiosity tended to be predictive of one or the other of the two primary drinking measures. Meaning Seeking and prior AA involvement predicted PDA 3 years later, and Religiosity was associated with less drinking intensity at 3 years. In addition to Self-efficacy Temptation minus Confidence, Confidence alone was also associated with better drinking outcomes at 1 and 3 years. Both general Motivation and alcohol-specific Readiness to Change predicted drinking outcomes at 1 and 3 years.

In the Aftercare arm, where drinking outcomes were measured only during the first year of follow-up, there were fewer prognostic variables. Self-efficacy Temptation minus Confidence was predictive of both PDA and DDD. Males drank more often and more intensely than females when they drank. Alcohol Involvement was associated with more DDD. The dissimilarity between the strength and kind of prognostic indicators in the two study arms supports the conclusion that assessments taken at the beginning of an outpatient treatment are more informative than those taken at the completion of intensive treatment just prior to the initiation of aftercare.

Client attributes also varied in their importance as prognostic indicators over time. Those associated with better drinking outcomes during treatment were not necessarily those associated with outcomes in the year following treatment. Thus, the clinician cannot assume that those doing better during treatment will also continue to do better following treatment. This finding also supports the importance of attending to what happens to the client in the post-treatment environment (Moos et al., 1990). It is of further interest that client attributes were generally better predictors of 3-year outcomes than of 1-year outcomes. Specifically, greater Alcohol Involvement, Meaning Seeking, and Prior Engagement in Alcoholics Anonymous were all prognostic of drinking outcomes 3 years after treatment, but not at 1 year.

Several variables previously reported to have prognostic value were not predictive of outcomes in this study. Most noteworthy, commonly shared pessimism regarding outcomes of antisocial and sociopathic clients (Hesselbrock et al., 1984) was not supported. Over the long term, these clients did no better or worse than the rest of the population. Because therapist optimism is itself associated with better outcomes (Leake & King, 1977), unwarranted pessimism about the chances for recovery in sociopathic clients should be re-evaluated (Longabaugh et al., 1994a). More generally, indices of psychiatric impairment (i.e., Axis I concurrent diagnosis and Addiction Severity Index (ASI) Psychiatric Severity) did not have prognostic value. Clients with or without concomitant psychological problems fared similarly on drinking outcomes in these alcohol-focused treatments. Levels of Cognitive Impairment also failed to predict client outcomes; more cognitively impaired clients fared just as well as those with less impairment.

Finally, several variables predicted outcome in the direction opposite to what would be anticipated from prior research. Poorer prognosis is often expected with greater Alcohol Involvement and Alcohol Dependence, Type B alcoholism, and with poorer Social Functioning. Clients who might have been expected to have poorer prognoses on the basis of these variables instead fared somewhat better in Project MATCH treatments. It must be remembered, however, that each predictor variable accounted for only a small proportion of outcome variance. As has been reported by other investigators (Moos et al., 1990), client pre-treatment characteristics do not, in fact, determine most of what happens in treatment outcome.

What about Alcoholics Anonymous involvement?

Because involvement in AA is relatively common among people in treatment for alcohol problems, it should be considered as a possible influence on treatment outcomes. In Project MATCH, 64% of Outpatients and 92% of Aftercare clients had had at least some exposure to AA before treatment. Many were at least somewhat involved in AA during and after treatment, particularly those assigned to the TSF treatment and clients in the Aftercare arm of the trial. In all three treatment conditions, AA involvement during the trial was predictive of better outcomes, and it appeared to have a particularly protective effect for clients with high Support for Drinking.

One misinterpretation of these findings must be noted: Project MATCH specifically does not support the conclusion that *instead* of going to treatment all one needs to do is attend AA. The TSF therapy was a well-structured, therapist-administered treatment. Even when AA involvement was taken into account, participation in TSF continued to predict significant variance in outcomes. Other studies have shown substantial outcome differences between treated clients and those only referred to AA (e.g., Walsh et al., 1991). What Project MATCH data do show is a positive relationship between AA involvement and abstinence, particularly among clients in the TSF treatment condition. Nevertheless, excellent outcomes also occur for many clients with no AA involvement.

Did findings vary across sites?

An interesting and unusual aspect of Project MATCH is the fact that the same study was repeated at five Aftercare and five Outpatient sites. In essence, the same study was done ten times with different client populations in nine different locations. The purpose of this, of course, was to increase confidence in the combined findings as generalizable across sites.

In the process, it was discovered that the same study would have come to rather different conclusions had it been conducted at only one or another of the sites. Although there were few striking differences in outcomes of the three treatments when all sites were combined, there were some sites at which clients fared quite differently depending upon the treatment to which they were randomly assigned. The direction of these differences was not consistent. Each of the three treatments had at least one site at which it did better than the other two, and at least one site at which its outcomes compared unfavorably with the others. Thus, depending upon which of the sites was conducting the study, a single site would have concluded that CBT was superior, or that TSF was best, or that, in general, clients assigned to MET had better outcomes. Each of these conclusions would, in the larger picture, have been misleading, and yet the fact stands that, at some sites, clients in one treatment did fare better. Whatever the reasons, the relative efficacy of different treatments appears to vary across sites at which they are tested.

When we detected overall matching effects, we also tested them to see whether they held up in both (Aftercare and Outpatient) arms of the trial. None of them did. This means that matches observed in one treatment setting may not apply at another.

Finally, there were interesting differences between outcomes for clients treated at outpatient sites, and those given aftercare following prior residential or day treatment. Although the Aftercare clients had had more severe problems on nearly every dimension studied, they also showed substantially better outcomes when compared with Outpatients given the same treatments in Project MATCH. The reasons for this are unclear. Aftercare clients were, in a sense, more self-selected because they had already completed a course of intensive treatment and were, by enrolling, signing up for 12 more weeks of Outpatient care. Aftercare clients also tended to enter Project MATCH already abstinent, giving them a head-start that they retained throughout the trial. Clients in the two arms of the trial differed from each other in many ways, and it may be that such pre-existing differences (such as greater severity and 'hitting bottom' among Aftercare clients) accounted for variations in outcome. It is also possible that the combination of prior interventions and Project MATCH treatments accounted for the better outcomes observed for Aftercare clients.

What can be concluded from Project MATCH?

The clearest surprise of Project MATCH was the modest support we found for matching clients to rather different, individually delivered treatments on the basis of clients' pre-treatment characteristics. To summarize the matching hypotheses that were supported:

- TSF was more effective than one or both of the other treatments with: (a) Outpatient clients without additional psychopathology, (b) Outpatients with high social support for continued drinking, (c) Aftercare clients high in alcohol dependence, and, to a lesser extent, (d) clients high in Meaning Seeking.

- MET was more effective than the other treatments for Outpatients high in anger.
- CBT was more effective than TSF with Aftercare clients low in alcohol dependence.

The magnitude of differences in the larger of these matching effects is sufficient to be clinically meaningful (e.g., differences of 10% to 17% in relapse rate or days abstinent). Keeping the bigger picture in mind, however, clients generally did quite well in any of the three treatment methods. One interpretation of this is that one need not feel greatly apologetic if offering only one of these approaches.

It is important, however, to avoid premature closure for the idea of offering an array of different approaches to which clients can be matched. Study design characteristics such as the extensive and frequent assessment of clients may have reduced the possibility of producing matching effects. Another possible explanation is that our matching hypotheses were insufficiently developed to specify the set of conditions under which matching would and would not occur. Moreover, Project MATCH was designed to test matching occurring from the pairing of single client attributes with one or the other of these three individually delivered treatments. It may be that matching among these three treatments will be clinically useful only when pertinent clinical profiles can be identified. From a broader perspective, there are many forms and aspects of treatment not tested here, such as pharmacotherapies, group therapies, different treatment settings, and different kinds of therapists. There may be meaningful matches between client characteristics and these attributes of treatment. Lastly, from a clinical perspective, for each treatment approach there are clients who find that approach unappealing, and the availability of options may help to retain them in treatment.

What about treatment for alcohol problems?

Project MATCH was not designed to test the hypothesis that treatment is better than no treatment. Its primary focus was on discovering which clients fared best in each of the three treatments offered, all of which were expected to be beneficial. The random assignment of treatment-seeking clients to receive or not to receive help would have been ethically unacceptable to virtually all of the clinical facilities that collaborated in Project MATCH, and would have threatened both the feasibility and the generalizability of the trial itself. The superiority of some alcohol treatments to other and briefer interventions has been demonstrated amply in a large body of clinical trials (Hester & Miller, 1995).

It is clear, however, that major improvements occurred relatively rapidly during the course of all three treatments, and persisted for at least 3 years afterward. On the whole, outcomes after the four-session MET were quite similar to those for the two 12-session treatments. This is consistent with a larger literature showing few differences when problem drinkers are randomly assigned to briefer versus longer treatments (Miller & Hester, 1986b; Bien et al., 1993). This comparability of outcomes held across the spectrum of problem severity; that is, the severity of alcohol problems did not interact with these treatments.

Project MATCH was the first randomized trial to compare a well-controlled Twelve Step-based treatment with other approaches. It is noteworthy, therefore, that the TSF therapy was associated throughout the trial with outcomes at least as favorable overall as those for MET and CBT. At various times and on certain measures, TSF clients fared significantly better. These modest differences were attributable to a higher rate of TSF clients maintaining complete continuous abstinence. Some of the observed matching effects also favored TSF over one or both of the other two approaches. In sum, TSF clearly deserves a place among treatments for alcohol problems.

Although total and continuous abstinence is too severe a standard for success, Project MATCH data do point to abstinence as a central outcome measure for research with alcohol-dependent, treatment-seeking clients. The PDA (versus drinking) was a good marker of other outcomes, and it was on this variable that most treatment differences were observed. Matching and therapist effects that were manifested on the intensity (DDD) measure were almost always reflected on the PDA measure as well. Clients who drank moderately and without problems also tended to have many abstinent days.

Summary

The findings of Project MATCH are both encouraging and humbling. By even the most stringent methodology, most clients show substantial improvement after treatment. Three very different treatment methods were associated with similarly positive outcomes. Client traits, sometimes thought to bode ill for outcomes, did not prove to be significant prognostic factors; instead, malleable states such as motivation and social support were most predictive. AA involvement was associated with better outcomes. Yet Project MATCH also highlights what we do not know about treatment, including some things widely assumed to be true. Support was modest for the popular idea of matching clients to optimal treatments on the basis of their pre-treatment characteristics. Many previously reported 'matching' interactions were not replicated. The variability of treatment effects across sites suggests one reason for this non-replication. Even under the stringently controlled conditions of this trial, different sites, if isolated, would have come to different conclusions. For those who devote their lives to helping others recover from alcohol abuse and dependence, many questions remain unanswered.

13

Clinical and scientific implications of Project MATCH

NED L. COONEY, THOMAS F. BABOR, CARLO C. DICLEMENTE,
AND FRANCES K. DEL BOCA

Ten years in the making, Project MATCH set out to address one of the critical research questions of its time. This chapter reviews the implications of the matching findings, as well as other results of the trial, for clinicians, policy makers, and researchers. Despite the small number of matching effects observed, the findings suggest that clinical efficacy may be improved in some cases if clinicians take into account certain characteristics (trait anger, alcohol dependence, social support for drinking, and psychiatric severity) when choosing among the three Project MATCH therapies. Beyond matching, the findings concerning Alcoholics Anonymous attendance and prognostic factors have additional implications for clinical practice, as do the 'best practices' that were developed for the trial. Perhaps the greatest impact of Project MATCH lies in its effect on theoretical assumptions about the nature of the therapeutic process in alcoholism treatment, and how best to investigate it.

Project MATCH was designed to provide a rigorous test of the alcoholism treatment matching hypothesis. We hypothesized that alcoholics with certain characteristics would have better outcomes when provided with a specific type of psychotherapy that matched their individual needs. In addition to testing the matching hypothesis, Project MATCH provided an opportunity to compare the overall outcomes of treatment with Cognitive–Behavioral Therapy (CBT), Motivational Enhancement Therapy (MET), and Twelve Step Facilitation (TSF). Treatment process analyses were conducted to examine the impact of Alcoholics Anonymous (AA) meeting attendance, the therapeutic alliance, and therapist characteristics. The fact that this was a multisite study allowed us to examine whether or not our findings were consistent across a variety of residential and outpatient settings. What are the lessons learned from Project MATCH? This chapter reviews the results of the trial in terms of their implications for practitioners, policy makers, and researchers.

Treatment matching

The primary aim of Project MATCH was to test the treatment matching hypothesis. Four out of 21 hypothesized matching effects achieved acceptable levels of statistical significance. These significant interactions involved client Anger, Social Support for drinking, severity of Alcohol Dependence, and Psychiatric Severity. However, the matching effect sizes were modest at best, and no matching effect was significant across both the Outpatient and Aftercare arms of the trial. For example, one of the strongest matching results, based on alcohol dependence, was only significant in the Aftercare arm, where matched clients had approximately a 63% success rate, compared with a 49% success rate for mismatched clients and a 56% success rate for unmatched or randomly assigned clients. The matching results were further weakened because they were often inconsistent across outcome measures and across follow-up time periods. Even if one assumes some modest benefit from each of the four significant matching strategies, there is no clear way to determine a proper match when the multiple matching criteria yield conflicting treatment assignments. Taken together, the strength of evidence for treatment matching based on results of Project MATCH is weak due to small matching effects and inconsistent results. Nevertheless, there is no reason why the following matching suggestions should not yield small improvements in drinking outcomes if applied under the right clinical conditions (Project MATCH Research Group, 1998c). TSF is suggested for outpatient clients without additional psychopathology, for outpatients whose social networks support continued drinking, and for aftercare clients high in alcohol dependence. MET is suggested for outpatients high in anger. CBT is suggested for aftercare clients low in alcohol dependence.

Choice of therapy

The results of Project MATCH provide insight into three treatments that are of tremendous interest to the field of addiction treatment. Cognitive–behavioral therapies and motivational enhancement therapies have been the subject of numerous alcoholism treatment outcome studies. In contrast, very little research has been conducted on Twelve Step treatment approaches. Project MATCH provided a unique opportunity to compare a new intervention derived from the principles of AA with two empirically validated treatments developed in academic settings, one that focused on skills training (CBT), and the other on motivational enhancement (MET). Given the absence of robust matching effects, the results of Project MATCH raise the interesting clinical question: is any one of these therapies 'better' than the others? The answer to this seemingly simple question depends on the study arm (Outpatient or Aftercare), on the time period (during treatment, 1 year after treatment, or 3 years after treatment), on the outcome measure (e.g., Percent Days Abstinent (PDA), Continuous Abstinence, Alcohol-related Consequences, or Composite outcome) and, to some extent, the characteristics of clients. In general, there were no outcome differences among the three treatments in the Aftercare arm. In the Outpatient arm, however, some modest differences emerged. During the 12-week treatment phase, CBT and TSF clients drank less often than MET clients. MET clients were drinking on an average of 20 days throughout the 90-day treatment phase, compared with 15 days for CBT and TSF clients. On a Composite outcome measure, more than 40% of CBT and TSF clients were classified as either abstinent or drinking moderately without problems, compared with 28% of MET clients.

Treatment differences faded among Outpatients in the year after treatment. No enduring clinically significant differences were found among treatments on measures of the frequency, intensity, and negative consequences of drinking. However, 24% of clients reported continuous abstinence throughout the year after treatment in the TSF condition, compared with 15% for CBT and 14% for MET. Abstinence rates in the Outpatient sample 3 years after treatment continued to favor TSF, with 36% reporting abstinence, compared with 24% for CBT and 27% for MET.

Thus, if one is asked to select only one of the three Project MATCH treatments for use across a range of clients, no recommendation can be made for the aftercare context. In an outpatient setting, however, CBT or TSF is recommended for limiting drinking and negative consequences during treatment. All three treatments were roughly equivalent on most measures after treatment, except that TSF produced higher total abstinence rates. TSF would thus be the treatment of choice to achieve long-term total abstinence in outpatient settings.

The favorable TSF outcomes in the Outpatient arm were somewhat surprising to the investigators. CBT and MET had both been evaluated in outcome studies, which showed them to be more effective than alternative therapies, whereas little research had been done using treatments based on the Twelve Steps. One lesson of Project MATCH is that an absence of empirical support for a treatment does not necessarily mean that the treatment is ineffective. It should be reiterated, however, that TSF is not the same as AA, although AA is a major element of the therapy.

The relative lack of differences among the three types of treatment suggests that each of them contains universal or nonspecific elements of effective therapy. What are these universal elements? Project MATCH provides some intriguing clues to the answer. First, the dramatic onset of abstinence during the early stage of treatment in the Outpatient arm suggests that the decision to initiate an episode of treatment allows many clients to mobilize a considerable amount of skill, motivation, and social network support for abstinence. This point is underscored by the strong prognostic effects of client motivation. In comparison to the initial mobilization of resources, the type of therapy, the characteristics of the therapist, and the match among client, therapy, and therapist may account for much less of the positive treatment effect than formerly believed. The clinical implications of this finding go beyond the more subtle distinctions that can be used to guide choice of treatment. They suggest that the value of having different types of therapy is not necessarily in their individual superiority or matching potential, but rather in their ability to convince clients that they are likely to benefit if they make the decision to begin therapy. Thus, a key ingredient to the success of any therapy may be its ability to attract clients and generate enthusiasm among therapists and program managers.

Another implication of these findings is that access to treatment may be as important as the type of treatment available to people with alcohol problems. If most treatments are similar in their effectiveness, the real value of having an array of treatments available is to promote healthy competition for the wide variety of people who would benefit from any treatment, but who would be more attracted to one because of reputation, convenience, or personal preference.

Finally, it is also possible that each of the three treatments has one or more unique elements that promote favorable outcomes, and that some combination of these features might provide an optimal psychosocial intervention.

Outpatient versus Aftercare treatment

There were dramatic differences in outcomes between clients treated in the Outpatient and Aftercare arms of Project MATCH. To illustrate the differences, outcome was classified as a 'success' when a client reported no heavy drinking or alcohol-related negative consequences in the preceding 3-month time period. Outcome was classified as a 'failure' when a client reported any heavy drinking and/or consequences in the 3-month time period. As described in Chapter 8, 27% more clients had successful outcomes during the treatment phase in the Aftercare arm than in the Outpatient arm. This impressive Aftercare advantage dissipated after treatment, but remained at 10% 1 year later.

It is possible that better outcomes in the Aftercare arm were due to the intensive treatment received in residential settings prior to the initiation of Project MATCH Aftercare therapies. However, this interpretation is not the only logical explanation for these findings. Clients were not randomized to study arms, and were recruited into the study using different procedures in each arm. Aftercare clients were recruited while they were enrolled in intensive, mostly inpatient, treatment programs. Outpatient clients came directly into Project MATCH therapies without prior intensive treatment except, in some cases, a brief detoxification. The comparison of Outpatient and Aftercare outcomes is confounded by the fact that Aftercare clients were admitted to the study only if they had successfully completed the intensive phase of treatment. This may have provided a motivational hurdle leading to exclusion of less-motivated clients. Because this exclusion process did not exist in the Outpatient arm, it is impossible to conclude that the 'respite' that was provided by the prior treatment of Aftercare clients was responsible for their superior outcomes. Nevertheless, there is evidence that intensive residential treatment may exert just this kind of a positive effect (Monahan & Finney, 1996), suggesting that residential programs followed immediately by additional aftercare treatment may produce outcomes that are superior to a single episode of outpatient treatment alone. It should also be noted that residential care may be recommended for reasons other than the enhancement of long-term outcomes. At times, it may be necessary to remove alcoholics from their immediate environment for medical, social, or psychiatric reasons. Although there has been a shift in the USA away from residential programs toward lower-intensity outpatient treatment, intensive programs might afford an initial impetus to sobriety that can be sustained in subsequent aftercare treatment. However, without further research and a more thorough analysis of the cost-effectiveness of prior intensive care, these observations remain highly speculative. Finally, Project MATCH treatments need to be adapted to real-world clinical settings to determine if efficacy in a controlled clinical trial translates into effectiveness in the community.

Alcoholics Anonymous attendance

One of the more significant clinical implications of the trial concerns the relationship among TSF, AA attendance, and outcome. In the USA, and increasingly in many other countries, the Twelve Step approach and the use of mutual support networks have become major features of a community's organized response to alcohol-related problems, particularly in treating people with alcohol dependence. Although the TSF treatment used in Project MATCH differs from AA in several respects, the findings described in Chapters 7, 8, and 11 provide insights into the mechanisms of action that account for the apparent success of AA. Project MATCH is perhaps the first study to effectively manipulate the amount of AA affiliation through the successful implementation of TSF. The findings suggest that AA affiliation can be increased by TSF, and that increased involvement in AA is associated with long-term sobriety. According to data presented in Chapters 7 and 8, Twelve Step approaches and AA seem to promote sobriety, not because they inspire a spiritual awakening in people who have lost meaning in life after they 'hit bottom,' but rather because they provide an alternative social network for people whose environment strongly supports their drinking (Longabaugh et al., 1998). However, AA may not be the most effective avenue of recovery for all alcoholics. The findings indicate that TSF worked best for Outpatients with pro-drinking social networks, and for Aftercare patients with high levels of alcohol dependence. Clients without these characteristics fared better in MET and CBT. The findings also provide insights into the timing and amount of AA involvement. TSF increased AA involvement during the 12-week treatment phase, but its influence seemed to persist even in the absence of active AA attendance after treatment.

To the extent that TSF enhanced AA involvement, especially during the active treatment phase, and that AA involvement was associated with improved outcomes far beyond the facilitation period, the findings of Project MATCH vindicate conventional wisdom that formal treatment can be enhanced by active collaboration with AA. But the findings go beyond conventional wisdom to suggest that AA, and perhaps other mutual-help organizations, need to be engaged during a critical period when the alcoholic is most motivated to take action in favor of recovery. If

the opportunity is missed during treatment to develop an active involvement with AA, it is much less likely that AA will exert its beneficial effects
in both the short term and the long term. From a policy perspective, the
findings of a reciprocal relationship between AA and formal treatment
indicate that both types of recovery programs need to be supported in the
context of a broader public health approach to tertiary prevention of
alcohol problems.

Prognostic characteristics

A few client characteristics strongly predicted Outpatient drinking outcomes across all three treatments. The most consistent predictor of outcome in the Outpatient arm was a measure of motivational Readiness to
Change. Greater Motivation predicted favorable Outpatient drinking outcomes during treatment as well as 1 and 3 years after treatment. This
measure was not prognostic for the Aftercare sample, perhaps because
these participants were assessed for motivation after involvement in several weeks of intensive treatment. A measure of Self-efficacy predicted
outcomes in both the Outpatient and Aftercare arms (DiClemente et al.,
2001a). Both Motivation and Self-efficacy are 'state' variables that are
thought to be changeable, holding out the hope that treatments that
modify these states could be more effective than treatments that do not.
These measures may be useful to identify clients most likely to benefit from
treatment, to assess progress in therapy, and to identify individuals at risk
for relapse.

Two other client characteristics predicted better outcomes: less social
support for drinking (in the Outpatient and Aftercare arms) and female
gender (in the Aftercare arm only). A number of characteristics that were
expected to predict unsuccessful outcome did not do so consistently,
including Psychiatric Severity, Sociopathy, Alcohol Involvement, Cognitive Impairment, Social Functioning, and Type B subtype (see Chapters 7
and 8). It appears that these characteristics and impairments do not doom
a client to continued drinking. This may be cause for optimism among
clinicians treating severely impaired clients.

Best practices

Another policy implication of Project MATCH is the lessons it offers for
the identification and dissemination of 'best practices.' Project MATCH

suggests that research-based procedures and practices, such as standardized diagnostic assessment, personalized feedback, therapist training in the use of manual-guided therapies, and deliberate facilitation into AA or other mutual-help organizations, may improve long-term outcomes.

Many treatment programs are overburdened by paperwork connected with reimbursement and administrative requirements, leaving little time to conduct a thorough diagnostic assessment of the client. The results of Project MATCH suggest that there are significant advantages to a well-conducted clinical assessment. Clients appreciate the time devoted to an understanding of their drinking problem. They can be motivated by the objective feedback produced by new assessment technologies, which provide the kind of normative information needed to address denial. Also, in programs offering a choice of therapeutic options, several of the simple assessments used in Project MATCH (i.e., trait Anger, Alcohol Dependence, Social Support for drinking) can lead to modest but valuable treatment matching effects.

Counselors and therapists who work with alcoholics are often guided by a combination of practical experience and prior training. The results of Project MATCH question some basic assumptions about the role of therapist characteristics in the process of recovery, and suggest ways in which therapists can improve their effectiveness. First, neither gender nor recovery status was associated with the success of treatment. The gender findings are consistent with other research (Gottheil et al., 1994; Sterling et al., 1998) indicating that patient–therapist gender matching does not increase treatment completion or improve outcomes. The finding that recovering alcoholics were no more effective than therapists not in recovery is somewhat at variance with the belief that recovering persons are more effective because they know alcoholism from their personal experience. The minimal contribution of therapist characteristics (except in the case of a few outliers who were considerably less effective than their counterparts) suggests that the training and supervision associated with the use of manual-guided therapies may have improved the overall effectiveness of treatment to the point where individual differences in skill or personality become relatively unimportant. With the increasing emphasis on professional credentialing, quality improvement, and accountability standards, these findings indicate that treatments can be standardized and often improved by the use of manual-guided therapies. Nevertheless, the experience of Project MATCH and other research (McLellan et al., 1997) suggests that the manual-guided treatments need to include components for clients with differing problems, allowing for some tailoring (matching) of treatments to client characteristics and practical needs.

Based upon the findings presented in Chapter 10, therapists need to pay attention to where the client is in his or her own personal process of change and to seek opportunities to facilitate that process. Clearly, more attention to client motivation is needed, particularly among outpatient clients (DiClemente et al., 2001b). Researchers and practitioners have been echoing this call over the past several years (Miller & Rollnick, 1991; DiClemente et al., 1992; Simpson et al., 1995; DiClemente & Scott, 1997; Miller & Heather, 1998). More focus on relapse prevention activities, both within and outside of the therapy session, is also needed. Although researchers have discovered more and more about the relapse process, preventing relapse continues to be a significant challenge (Carroll, 1996; Dimeff & Marlatt, 1998). Finally, clinicians should allow clients to talk about how tempted they are to drink and assess the level of efficacy to perform the various target behaviors needed for recovery. Allowing the client to voice uncertainty and lack of efficaciousness can provide an opportunity to influence the client's process of change at a critical point in recovery.

One area where the results of Project MATCH are consistent with conventional wisdom and with professional practice is in the value of coordinating formal treatment with the mutual-help community. In the USA, and in many other countries throughout the world, over 2 million recovering alcoholics can be found on any given day participating in mutual-help groups such as AA. Although not all recovering persons need or will benefit from these groups, the results of Project MATCH show that the initial gains realized in formal treatment can be enhanced and prolonged if strong encouragement is given to the initiation of an aftercare plan that includes the support of mutual-help organizations.

Implications for theory and research

The findings raise some important questions about theory and method in the exploration of treatment matching. Project MATCH provided ample opportunity to test some basic assumptions about how treatment works and why some alcoholics benefit from treatment and others do not. Although there were predictable reductions in drinking following treatment, there were few indications that one treatment was more effective than the others, regardless of the type of therapy or its intensity. When matching effects were observed, the causal chain analyses indicated that, in most cases, the therapy was not operating according to the predicted relationship between client characteristics and the therapeutic process elements (Longabaugh & Wirtz, 2001). For example, MET was effective for clients who had high levels of anger, but the therapy did not produce the changes in anger that were expected according to the mechanisms suggested by cognitive–behavioral and motivational theory. Ironically, the therapy with the least empirical support from previous research (i.e., TSF) seemed to work, in part, because of the social mechanism of action that has long been part of AA lore. By connecting alcoholics with a fellowship of recovering people who support abstinence, TSF was differentially effective for alcoholics who had social networks that supported heavy drinking. Not only did TSF succeed in strengthening the bond with AA, but also higher AA involvement was associated with better drinking outcomes 3 years after the end of treatment for Outpatient clients who needed it most, i.e., those with social networks that encouraged drinking (Longabaugh et al., 1998).

However, further examination of an alternative causal chain, this one suggesting a process whereby TSF produces spiritual changes connected with the search for a higher meaning in life, did not confirm the predicted association. Thus, Project MATCH provides not only a clear test of alternative theories, it also indicates the importance of studying basic assumptions as well as the more practical effects of treatment. Without knowledge of why a particular treatment works, both researchers and clinicians are doomed to operate in a world governed by either clinical intuition or blind empiricism. Neither approach does justice to the needs of alcoholics.

An important theoretical implication of these findings is their potential for understanding the active ingredients of treatment. The findings were ambiguous with regard to MET and CBT, but the causal chain analyses of TSF (Chapter 7) indicated that social support for drinking is a particularly important determinant of the long-term sobriety of alcoholics with networks that encourage drinking. These findings demonstrate the value of theory in guiding both research and clinical practice. If the essential elements of a treatment can be identified, it may be possible to strengthen those elements and reduce the resources and costs devoted to superfluous elements. This conclusion, however, is predicated on the assumption that different treatments work because of distinct, non-overlapping mechanisms, instead of through common mechanisms, such as empathy, an effective working alliance between the therapist and the client, a desire to get better, the alcoholic's inner resources to overcome alcohol dependence, a supportive social network, and the provision of a culturally appropriate solution to a socially defined problem.

Project MATCH provided no theoretical support for specific mechanisms behind CBT and MET, and this is consistent with the results of other research. Morgenstern and Longabaugh (2000), for example, found that numerous studies have failed to provide even presumptive support for the mediational hypothesis that CBT works through its effects on coping skills. If CBT is effective, but not for the reasons postulated by its developers, it may indicate that nonspecific factors, such as the therapist's empathy or the therapeutic alliance, are more important to an understanding of therapeutic change.

Despite the high expectations that Project MATCH would provide definitive answers to the most pressing questions about treatment matching, the findings suggest that no single study, regardless of its cost or its scope, is capable of addressing all relevant issues in relation to clinical practice, theory testing, and policy choices. A full analysis of the matching question, given the benefit of hindsight, would now seem to require the more systematic study of a full range of treatments over a full range of client severity over the full range of the drinking career. Although Project MATCH provides important information about the efficacy of matching with different short-term psychotherapies, it may be more fruitful in the future to study matching in larger populations at the level of communities or treatment systems, where a larger range of settings and therapeutic interventions can be evaluated with a broader range of alcohol-dependent clients over a more representative span of their drinking careers. A major step in this direction has already been taken by Ouimette et al. (1998), whose study of TSF and CBT in several large treatment programs produced results similar to those of Project MATCH.

It should also be recognized that research methods as well as the research questions they serve are conditioned by historical circumstances and cultural assumptions. History will tell whether Project MATCH fairly addressed an eminently sensible research question with the most appropriate scientific methodology, or whether it represented the limited priorities of a particular culture during a particular historical period. It is the belief of the Project MATCH Research Group that the study's findings will endure as a definitive answer to the matching question, even as the methods and theory that developed out of the trial will continue to stimulate new research in other directions.

Far from disconfirming the matching hypothesis, Project MATCH may well have uncovered some critical mechanisms of treatment efficacy, and suggested a radical alternative to the assumptions of clinical science that have guided its basic approach to theory testing. In many respects, Project MATCH was predicated on assumptions of the 'technology model' of psychotherapy, which bear resemblance to the classic 'Medical Model,' in which specific treatment interventions or ingredients are directed at the specific disease process or biological deficiencies that are assumed to be responsible for the patient's symptoms. Although evidence for some specific causal mechanisms was found to underlie successful treatment matching (e.g., social support, dependence severity), the effects were not powerful or consistent enough to recommend major changes in the way clients are assigned to treatment in short-term psychotherapy. Nevertheless, the rapid and substantial decline in drinking that followed the client's engagement in treatment raises fascinating questions about how treatment influences drinking behavior.

There is an old adage that says: 'If left untreated, a cold will last one week, but if treated with the latest cold remedy, it will be gone in seven days.' A related adage says: 'God heals and the doctor takes the credit.' The same kinds of conventional wisdom have been applied to the treatment of alcohol problems, implying that, like many illnesses and behavior problems, alcohol dependence will eventually be resolved without direct intervention. Modern medicine, rejecting the idea that treatment is merely a placebo, has certainly demonstrated success in applying the medical or technology model to infectious and communicable diseases as well as the application of surgical and chemical interventions. But this model may have its limits in the study and understanding of biobehavioral conditions like alcohol dependence. Perhaps the experience gained with Project MATCH will redirect attention by scientists and clinicians to the more complex interaction between patients and treatment that heretofore has been more the interest of anthropologists and sociologists than of psychologists and psychiatrists.

This is not to suggest that the outcomes observed following Project MATCH's three treatments can be explained by some kind of placebo effect, by spontaneous remission of alcohol dependence, or by 'regression to the mean' as alcohol problems wax and wane. Although some of the improvement observed after the onset of treatment can surely be explained as the natural course of alcoholism, which is a chronic relapsing condition with periods of sobriety intervening between periods of problem drinking, it is likely that formal treatment serves to accelerate the natural recovery process by providing the resources necessary to stop now rather than later. What may be required even more than the specific components of a therapeutic intervention is the belief on the part of both the patient and the therapist that this particular treatment is likely to be effective.

In the future, researchers may therefore be advised to focus more upon how treatments interact with the client process of intentional behavioral change. Treatment comparisons would be more likely to identify signifi-cant differences if they could demonstrate that they reliably produce differential effects on the client's motivation and self-efficacy. At issue is whether any treatment could enhance or interfere with what appears to be a common pathway of changing drinking behavior. If we have treatments that can demonstrate differential effects on motivation, efficacy, or coping activities, then we might be able to more effectively examine treatment differences, causal mechanisms, and even potential matching effects. As this and other studies have shown, treatments can have very different assumptions, theoretically distinct rationales, and clearly different stra-tegies without producing different results. Often clients report similar levels of satisfaction and types of personal experience after having been in very different treatments (Sloane et al., 1975). A number of years ago, Jerome Frank (1976) wrote that psychotherapy should be understood in the context of a more general process that he labeled 'persuasion and healing.' In his view, the nonspecific elements of trust, belief, and hope are responsible for creating change. Similarly, Carl Rogers (1957) indicated that therapist empathy, genuineness, and warmth set the stage for change wherein the individual is enabled to develop greater congruence between the real and the ideal selves. Both of these perspectives focus on the therapist as healer or facilitator of a rather generic client change process that is not behavior specific. Perhaps the next frontier in psychotherapy research is to understand more fully the client process of intentional behavioral change and how therapists influence that process.

Research related to therapists should include what the therapist can do to interfere with as well as to potentiate the process of change. There have been many myths about who therapists should be and what they should do. The Project MATCH data counter some of these myths. Therapists do not need to be recovering from addiction, matched on gender (except possibly among female Outpatients in TSF), or have many years of experi-ence to be effective. However, individual therapists can have deleterious effects on their clients in terms of drinking outcomes. We should study not only the successful therapists, but also the least successful ones in order to understand what they do that promotes or interferes with change. There are some interesting leads in our analyses of the therapist data that need additional research. To ignore these findings would counter the dictum 'primum, non nocere' – first, do no harm.

Methodological implications

Some of the most interesting findings to emerge from Project MATCH were secondary to the major focus of the investigation, which was designed to study treatment matching rather than treatment efficacy, therapist effects, or the effectiveness of AA. Given the small amount of matching that was observed, it might be argued that the conditions surrounding the implementation of a large-scale clinical trial (such as videotaped therapy sessions, hours of diagnostic assessments, frequent follow-up interviews with research staff) may have diluted or obscured any matching effects that might be manifested under more typical clinical conditions. This is the classic trade-off between internal and external validity. The more a rigorous research design improves the chances of drawing valid causal inferences, the more it may limit the generalizability of the conclusions. Nevertheless, without the ability to make unequivocal causal inferences, a major clinical trial like Project MATCH would be a meaningless exercise. Also, to suggest that intensive diagnostic assessment or frequent research interviews, rather than alcohol treatment, is the main reason for the observed reductions in drinking is to argue that treatment effects are so lacking in specificity that therapy is irrelevant, even as a culturally sanctioned excuse for choosing sobriety.

Project MATCH in many respects constituted a new, mission-oriented approach to alcoholism treatment research, one that provides important lessons for those who are interested in designing, implementing, and evaluating new ways to reduce the societal costs and human suffering of people with alcohol dependence. In the process, new clinical research technologies (such as urn randomization), new statistical approaches to longitudinal data analysis, and new assessment procedures were applied to the study of alcoholism treatment. It also created major challenges for the collection of data from multiple sites, and the standardization of treatment and research protocols across different sites. Some have questioned the wisdom of such an extensive collaborative undertaking, given the total costs of the trial (approximately $28 million) and the time it took to reach fruition (10 years). But, in light of the number of clients studied (1726), the extent of the follow-up evaluation (up to 39 months), the scientific publications (over 90 scientific articles, books, monographs, and commentaries), and other products (treatment manuals, methodological innovations) that were produced, the cost may not have been excessive. Clinical research studies are expensive to conduct, and Project MATCH was no more expensive per patient than other clinical trials. Large-scale trials have an important role to play in the development of clinical science. They are needed just as much as small-scale trials, especially when smaller, less methodologically rigorous studies produce findings that are intriguing but insufficient to dictate treatment policy.

Finally, it should be noted that the randomized clinical trial, though rightfully considered the standard methodology for evaluating treatment efficacy, should not be the only approach to the investigation of treatment matching. Prospective observational cohort studies can approximate the results of randomized clinical trials if they are based on the same design principles and patient assembly procedures (Horwitz et al., 1990).

Research using less rigorous, quasi-experimental designs has shown that matching to existing services produces findings similar to those observed in Project MATCH (Ouimette et al., 1999).

Matching research is perhaps the most challenging form of clinical investigation, conceptually, methodologically, and practically. But this is not to say that matching research should be abandoned. On the contrary, considerable progress has been made in the areas of conceptualization, measurement of key variables, the specification of treatment, the development of research designs, and the assessment of treatment outcomes. Taken together, these developments offer promise that treatment matching research could provide significant findings relevant to the evaluation of current services and the design of new types and systems of treatment.

Summary

In summary, perhaps the real implications of Project MATCH, in the words of one observer (Ashton, 1999, p. 15), lie 'more in its unanticipated findings than in what it set out so painstakingly to prove – less in matching treatment technologies to patient variables, more in the human touch and doing whatever you do well.' This applies as much to clinical practice as it does to scientific research. Ten years in the making, Project MATCH is best understood not as a series of isolated reports, but as a complex intellectual undertaking that attempted to address one of the critical research questions of its time. If the findings reported in this volume give an unexpected and not always flattering answer to the matching question, so are they likely to establish new insights, new standards, and new questions to pursue.

Appendix

Personnel and facilities affiliated with Project MATCH

This appendix provides a comprehensive listing of the personnel and facilities affiliated with Project MATCH between 1989 and 1999. The key at the end of the appendix provides definitions of the abbreviations used to designate people's roles in the project, their academic degrees, and professional certifications.

National Institute on Alcohol Abuse and Alcoholism

Richard K. Fuller, MD, Director, Division of Clinical and Prevention Research
John P. Allen, PhD, Chief, Treatment Research Branch, Project Officer
Margaret E. Mattson, PhD, Staff Collaborator

Clinical Research Units

William R. Miller, PhD, P.I., and J. Scott Tonigan, PhD, co-P.I., University of New Mexico, Albuquerque, NM

Gerard J. Connors, PhD, P.I., and Robert G. Rychtarik, PhD, co-P.I., Research Institute on Addictions, Buffalo, NY

Carrie L. Randall, PhD, P.I., and Raymond F. Anton, MD, co-P.I., Medical University of South Carolina and Veterans Affairs Medical Center, Charleston, SC

Ronald M. Kadden, PhD, P.I., University of Connecticut School of Medicine, Farmington, CT, and Mark D. Litt, PhD, co-PI, University of Connecticut School of Dental Medicine and School of Medicine, Farmington, CT

Carlo C. DiClemente, PhD, P.I., and Joseph Carbonari, EdD, co-P.I., University of Houston, Houston, TX

Allen Zweben, DSW, P.I. and Ron Cisler, PhD, co-P.I., Center for Addiction and Behavioral Research, University of Wisconsin, Milwaukee, WI

Richard H. Longabaugh, EdD, P.I., and Robert L. Stout, PhD, co-P.I., Brown University, Providence, RI

Dennis Donovan, PhD, co-P.I. and R. Dale Walker, MD, P.I. University of Washington and Seattle Veterans Affairs Medical Center, Seattle, WA

Ned L. Cooney, PhD, P.I., West Haven Veterans Affairs Medical Center and Yale University School of Medicine, New Haven, CT

Coordinating Center

Thomas F. Babor, PhD, P.I., and Frances K. Del Boca, PhD, co-P.I., University of Connecticut, Farmington, CT
Bruce J. Rounsaville, MD, P.I., and Kathleen M. Carroll, PhD, co-P.I., Yale University, New Haven, CT

Consultants

Larry Muenz, PhD, Gaithersburg, MD
Philip Wirtz, PhD, George Washington University, Washington, DC
L.J. Wei, PhD, Harvard University, Cambridge, MA

Collaborating Investigators

Su Bailey, PhD, Veterans Affairs Medical Center–Houston, and Department of Psychiatry, Baylor College of Medicine, Houston, TX
Kathleen Brady, PhD, MD, Institute of Psychiatry, Medical University of South Carolina, Charleston, SC
Daniel R. Kivlahan, PhD, Veterans Affairs Medical Center, Seattle, and Department of Psychiatry and Behavioral Sciences, University of Washington School of Medicine, Seattle, WA
Ted D. Nirenberg, PhD, Roger Williams Medical Center and Brown University, Providence, RI
Lauren A. Pate, MD, Veterans Affairs Medical Center–Houston, and Department of Psychiatry, Baylor College of Medicine, Houston, TX
Sandra Rasmussen, PhD, Southwood Community Hospital, Providence, RI
Ellie Sturgis, PhD, Medical University of South Carolina, Charleston, SC
Reid Hester, PhD, Center on Alcoholism, Substance Abuse, and Addictions, University of New Mexico, Albuquerque, NM

Collaborating Facilities

Care Unit Hospital of Kirkland, Kirkland, WA (Karen Porter-Frazier, RN, and Jan Bigby-Hanson, MSW)
Charleston County Substance Abuse Commission, Charleston, SC (Barbara Derrick, Executive Director)
CPC Greenbriar Hospital, Milwaukee, WI (Donald C. Fisher, MD)
DePaul Hospital, Milwaukee, WI (Brian E. Tugana, MD, MBA)
Fenwick Hall Hospital, Charleston, SC (John Magill, CEO)

Harris County Psychiatric Center, Houston, TX (Ken Krajewski, MD, and Terry Rustin, MD)

Ivanhoe Treatment Center, Milwaukee, WI (Marion R. Romberger)

Lawrence Center, Waukesha Memorial Hospital, Waukesha, WI (Fred Syrjanen, MS, CADC-III)

Medical University of South Carolina, Institute of Psychiatry, Charleston, SC (James C. Ballenger, MD, Director)

Metro Milwaukee Recovery Center, Milwaukee, WI (Steve Skowlund, MA, CADC-III)

Milwaukee Psychiatric Hospital, Wauwatosa, WI (Patty Priebe, RN)

Northwest General Hospital, Milwaukee, WI (Richard Hicks, BA)

Roger Williams General Hospital, Providence, RI (Ted Nirenberg, PhD)

Schick-Shadel Hospital, Seattle, WA (James W. Smith, MD, and Michael Olsson, MS)

Sinai Samaritan Hospital, Milwaukee, WI (Tom Johnston, MSW)

Southeastern Wisconsin Medical and Social Services, Milwaukee, WI (Lawrence Neuser, President)

Southwood Community Hospital, Norfolk, MA (Yolanda Landrau, RN, EdD, and Rhoda Stevens, RN, CAC)

Veterans Affairs Medical Center, Charleston, SC (Byron Adinoff, MD)

Veterans Affairs Medical Center, Houston, TX (Lauren Pate, MD, and Su Bailey, PhD)

Veterans Affairs Medical Center, Milwaukee, WI (Dennis Borski, MSW, and Jung-Ki Cho, MD)

Veterans Affairs Medical Center, Seattle, WA (Daniel R. Kivlahan, PhD)

Data Safety and Monitoring Board

Paul Cushman, Jr, MD, Department of Psychiatry, State University of New York, Stony Brook, NY

John Finney, PhD, Center for Health Care Evaluation, Program Evaluation and Resource Center (152), Department of Veteran Affairs, Menlo Park, CA

Ralph Hingson, ScD, Social Behavior and Sciences Section, Boston University School of Public Health, Boston, MA

James Klett, PhD, Bel Air, MD

Michael Townsend, PhD, Division of Substance Abuse, Cabinet for Human Research, Frankfort, KY

Project MATCH Research Personnel

ALBUQUERQUE: Robert J. Meyers, MS (P.C.); Andrea Anderson (S.A.); Lisa T. Arciniega, MS (R.A., P.C.); Francesca Ashcroft (C.I.); Janice Brown, Test/Retest Subject Coordinator; Brenda Carreon (S.A.); Janet C'de Baca (D.A.); Susanna Chang (R.A.); Demetrius Gonzales (C.I.); Randy Granger (S.A.); Anne

Hahn-Smith, MS (R.A.); Dina Hill (R.A.); Margaret Johnston (D.A.); Mary Kaven, PhD (R.A.); Lee Ann LeBrier (C.I.); Laura Little, MS (R.A.); Mayrem Musa (C.I.); Juanita Pasco (R.A.); HollyBeth Prince MA (D.A.); Ron Prince (D.A.); Dee Ann Quintana (A.A.); Stephanie Romero (C.I.); Pauline Sawyers, MS (R.A.); Natasha Slesnick-Jaderlund, MS (R.A.); Paige Spence (C.I.); Jim Story, MS (R.A.); Kamilla Willoughby (R.A.); Delilah Yao (A.A.)

BUFFALO: Kurt Dermen, PhD (P.C.); Claudia Casey, MBA (R.A.); Mark Duerr, MA (R.A.); Kim Haag, MA (R.A.); James Koutsky, MA (R.A.); Melissa Kulick, MS (R.A.); Cathy Lovejoy (R.A.); Deborah Ross, MS (R.A.); Anupama Sharma, MA (R.A.); Karen Steinberg, PhD (R.A.); Rachelle Strachar-Behm (R.A.); Mark Veronica (R.A.)

CHARLESTON: Angelica Thevos, MSW, ACSW (P.C.); Charleene Baxter, MSW (C.I.); Mary Ann Boyd (R.A.); Janice Brown, MA (D.A.); Bernadette Cooper (D.A.); Louise Hammes (R.A.); B.J. Harris (D.A.); Stacy Inabinett (R.A.); Kristen Jerger (R.A.); Antoinette M. Laster (D.A.); Penny Mills (R.A.); Tamara Reuter (D.A.); Kim Turner (R.A.); Becky Wood (R.A.)

FARMINGTON: Laura Ginther, PsyD (P.C.); Elise Kabela, PhD (P.C.); Amy Brener (R.A.); Deborah Busher (R.A.); Carol Kennedy (R.A.); Thad Kobus (R.A.); Pat Korner, RN, CARN, Medical Evaluation; Peter Manu, MD, Medical Evaluation; Tracey Meier (R.A.); Chris Napolitano (R.A.); Cheryl Pacyna, MA (R.A.); Sue Tomlinson (R.A.)

HOUSTON: Mary Marden Velasquez, PhD (P.C.); LaRay Adame, MA (R.A.); Allison Bruce (R.A.); Wendy Daigler (R.A.); Gaylyn Gaddy (R.A.); Tom Irwin (R.A.); Teresa King MA (R.A.); Rosario Montgomery, MA (R.A.); Lynn Oswald, MSN (R.A.); David Pena (R.A.); Jennifer Rothfleisch (R.A.); Kirk Von Stemberg (R.A.); Kelli Wright (R.A.)

MILWAUKEE: David Barrett, MS, CADC-III (P.C.); Michael Bauer, MSW (R.A.); Don Bennett (R.A.); Jean D'Amato (A.A.); Kris Dunlap, MEd (R.A.); Jean Gasvoda, MSW, CADC-III (R.A.); Kristin Hackl, MSW (R.A.); Fred Harvey, CADC-III, Intake Coordinator; Cherie Horan (R.A.); Nancy Jaegers, RN (R.A.); Angie Kessler, CADC (R.A.); Raymond Konz, MSW (R.A.); Carol Kozminiski (D.A.); Lorri Multer, MA (R.A.); Lisa Rindt (A.A.); Dawn Rolling (R.A.); Jody Schmidt, CADC (R.A.); Hope Schrader (R.A.); Mark Schwallie (R.A.); Dennis Shirk, CADC-III (R.A.); Chris Steigenberaer (R.A.); Denise Tomka (D.A.); Sheila Van Rixell, MS, CADC-III (R.A.); Sharon Weisensal (R.A.); Marguirite Woodfill, CADC-III (R.A.); Paul Zenisek, MSSW, CADC-III (R.A.)

PROVIDENCE: Christopher Rice, PhD (P.C./Co-Investigator); Kathleen Carty (R.A.); Nancy Cole, MA (C.I.); Katharine Dodae (C.I.); Lisa Freda (R.A.); Connie Lawson (R.A.); Bethany Letiecq (R.A.); Isabel McDevitt (A.A.); Marjorie McMahon (R.A.); Jerry Maske (R.A.); Racquel Pina (C.I.); Gina Rogirri (C.I.); Maureen Walsh (R.A.)

SEATTLE: David Rosengren, PhD (P.C.); Peg Wood, PhD (P.C.); Bonnie Allen,

QCDC (R.A.); Pamela Bakke (A.A.); Stephanie Ballasiotes, QCDC (R.A.); Molly Carney, MA (R.A.); Hackman Chan (D.A.); Laurie Deppinan (R.A.); Heidi Erickson (R.A.); Kristen Korell (R.A.); Patti Matestic (S.A.); Krista Mortensen (D.A.); Jane Tinker, PhD (R.A.); Ann Ward (S.A.); Karyn Wubbena, QCDC (R.A.)

WEST HAVEN: Priscilla Morse, MA (P.C.); Matthew Snow, PhD (P.C.); Elsa Bastone, PhD, Clinical Coordinator; Gerry Battista (R.A.); Tim Coffey (R.A.); Susan Devine (R.A.); Eric Pero (R.A.); Diane Walton (R.A.)

FARMINGTON COORDINATING CENTER: Bonnie McRee (P.C.); Meredith Weidenmann (P.C.); Suzanne Chorches (D.A.); Bradley Collins (D.A.); Anne McLaney, PhD (D.A.); Richard Mendola, PhD (C.P.); Cynthia Mohr (D.M.); Debbie Talamini (A.A.); Eva Vavrousek-Jakuba, PhD (D.A.); Janice Vendetti (D.M.); Penina Weisenberg (C.P.)

YALE COORDINATING CENTER: Heidi Behr (R.A.); Roseann Bisighini (R.A.), Kathryn Nuro, PhD (P.C.); Tami Frankforter (D.M.); Charla Nich, MS (D.A.); Joanne Corvino, MPH (R.A.)

National Institute on Alcohol Abuse and Alcoholism

Megan Columbus, Program Analyst; Joel Kirkpatrick, Computer Clerk; Rita Lehr, Senior Program Assistant; Veronica Wilson, Program Analyst

Project MATCH Therapy Personnel

COGNITIVE–BEHAVIORAL THERAPY (C.B.T.): Adam Jaffe, PhD; Daniel Keller, PhD; James Langenbucher, PhD; Georgeann Witte, PhD

MOTIVATIONAL ENHANCEMENT THERAPY (M.E.T.): Sharon Chappell, MSW; Catherine Nogas-Steinberg, MA

TWELVE STEP FACILITATION THERAPY (T.S.F.); Stuart Baker, MA, CAC; Joseph Nowinski, PhD; Charles Wilbur, MEd

OTHER THERAPY CONSULTANTS: Twelve Step manual writers: Joseph Nowinski, PhD, and Stuart Baker, MA, CAC; Hazelden Foundation: Pat Owen, PhD, Dan Anderson, PhD, and Fred Holmquist

Project MATCH Therapists

ALBUQUERQUE: Gina Civerolo, MA (C.B.T.); Molly Evanko, MA (T.S.F.); Joseph Bo Miller, MSW (M.E.T.); Henry Montgomery, MS (T.S.F.); Edward T. Nash, PhD (M.E.T.); Craig Noonan, MSW (C.B.T.); Gary Randolph (T.S.F.); Maurice Rodriguez (C.B.T.); Julianne West, MA (T.S.F.); Karla Whetstone, MA (T.S.F.)

BUFFALO: Rellie Boyd, CAC (T.S.F.); Cathleen Carter, PhD (C.B.T.); Joan Duquette, MS, CAC (T.S.F.); Andrea Lingenfelter, CAC (C.B.T.); Linda Meeker, CSW (M.E.T.); Kathleen Morinello, CAC (T.S.F.); Mary Schohn, PhD (C.B.T.); Mariela Shirley, PhD (C.B.T.); Jeremy Skinner, PhD (M.E.T.); Renee Wert, PhD (M.E.T.)

CHARLESTON: Sharon Becker, MSW, ACSW (C.B.T.); Donald Geddes, MEd, LPC (T.S.F.); Valerie Holmstrom, PhD (C.B.T.); Patricia Latham, RN, PhD (T.S.F.); Darlene Shaw, PhD (M.E.T.); Martha Tumblin, MEd, LISW (T.S.F.); L. Randolph Waid, PhD (M.E.T.)

FARMINGTON: Patricia Burke, RN, MSN (M.E.T.); Kathleen Chapman, MA (T.S.F.); Laura Ginther, PsyD (C.B.T.); Janet Mitchell Hall, RN, MS (M.E.T.); Janine K. Lasch, CAC/CDAC (T.S.F.); Christopher Penta, MA, NCC, CCMHC (C.B.T.); Aimee Perkins, MS (M.E.T.); Bernice Shaker, RN, MS, CS (M.E.T.); Arthur H. Woodard, Jr., MSW (T.S.F.)

HOUSTON: Deborah Collins, CADAC (T.S.F.); Douglas Gilbert, MA (M.E.T.); Sharon Gillam, LCDC (T.S.F.); John Green, LCDC (T.S.F.); Carol Katulich, MA, CADAC (T.S.F.); Elizabeth O'Connor, MA (C.B.T.); Ken Sewell, MA (C.B.T.); Julia Stauffer, MA (C.B.T.); Nanette Stephens, MA (M.E.T.); Angela Stotts, MA (M.E.T.); Norman Weeden, MA, CADAC (T.S.F.)

MILWAUKEE: Bertrand Berger, PhD (C.B.T.); Patricia Beilke, PhD (M.E.T.); Bonnie Bjodstrup, MSW (M.E.T.); Mark Dearth, CADC-III (T.S.F.); James Holifield, MSW (C.B.T.); Margie Pecus, MSW (T.S.F.); Karen Scholz, CADC-II (T.S.F.); Virginia Stoffel, MS, OTR (C.B.T.)

PROVIDENCE: John D'Agenais, MA, CAC (T.S.F.); Joan Ferguson, MA, CDP (T.S.F.); James Femey, CDP (M.E.T.); Robert D. Hawes, MS (M.E.T.); Jane Mitchell, MEd (C.B.T.); Ed O'Brien, MEd (C.B.T.); Moirna O'Rourke, MA (M.E.T.); David Stem, PsyD (C.B.T.)

SEATTLE: Kerry Bartlett, PhD (M.E.T.); Dennis Donovan, PhD (C.B.T.); Josephine Hadlock-King, MSW (M.E.T.); Jerry Hagen, MSW (T.S.F.); Deborah Hillman, MSW (C.B.T.); Patti Joyce, MA (M.E.T.); Priscilla MacKay, PhD (C.B.T.); Denise Pritzl, MSW (M.E.T.); Dwight Randolph, MA, MPA, QCDC (T.S.F.); George Thomas, MA, CCDC (T.S.F.)

WEST HAVEN: James E. Baker, MA, CAC (M.E.T.); Cheryl Gelernter, PhD (C.B.T.); Julie Jarvis, MA, CAC (C.B.T.); Richard Kantlehner, MA, CAC (T.S.F.); Les Martel, PhD (C.B.T.); Chris Salonia, CAC (T.S.F.); Carrie Schaffer, PhD (M.E.T.); Matt Snow, PhD (C.B.T.)

Key

Role in project	*Definition*
A.A.	Administrative Assistant
C.I.	Collateral Interviewer
C.P.	Computer Programmer
co-P.I.	Co-Principal Investigator
D.A.	Data Assistant
P.C.	Project Coordinator
P.I.	Principal Investigator
R.A.	Research Assistant/Associate
S.A.	Staff Assistant

Degrees / certification	*Definition*
ACSW	Academy Certified Social Worker
CAC	Certified Alcoholism Counselor
CADAC	Certified Alcohol and Drug Abuse Counselor
CADC	Certified Alcohol and Drug Counselor
CARN	Certified Addiction Registered Nurse
CCDC	Certified Chemical Dependence Counselor
CCMHC	Certified Clinical Mental Health Counselor
CDP	Certified in Data Processing
CEO	Chief Executive Officer
LCDC	Licensed Chemical Dependence Counselor
LISW	Licensed Independent Social Worker
LPC	Licensed Professional Counselor
MBA	Master of Business Administration
MD	Doctor of Medicine
MEd	Master of Education
MPA	Master of Public Administration
MPH	Master of Public Health
MS	Master of Science
MSN	Master of Science in Nursing
MSSW	Master of Science in Social Work
MSW	Master of Social Work
NCC	Nationally Certified Counselor
OTR	Occupational Therapist Registered
PhD	Doctor of Philosophy
PsyD	Doctor of Psychology
QCDC	Qualified Chemical Dependency Counselor
RN	Registered Nurse
ScD	Doctor of Science

References

Alcoholics Anonymous (1975) *Living Sober: Some Methods A.A. Members Have Used for Not Drinking.* New York: Alcoholics Anonymous World Services, Inc.

Alcoholics Anonymous (1976) *Alcoholics Anonymous (The Blue Book).* New York: Alcoholics Anonymous World Services, Inc.

Alcoholics Anonymous (1981) *Twelve Steps and Twelve Traditions.* New York: Alcoholics Anonymous World Services, Inc.

Alcoholics Anonymous (1997) *Alcoholics Anonymous 1996 Membership Survey.* New York: Alcoholics Anonymous World Services, Inc.

Allen, J.P. & Columbus, M. (eds) (1995) *Assessing Alcohol Problems: a Guide for Clinicians and Researchers.* Bethesda, MD: National Institute on Alcohol Abuse and Alcoholism.

Allen, J.P. & Kadden, R.M. (1995) Matching clients to alcohol treatments. In *Handbook of Alcoholism Treatment Approaches: Effective Alternatives*, ed. Hester, R.K. & Miller, W.R. Needham Heights, MA: Allyn and Bacon, 278–91.

American Psychiatric Association (1987) *Diagnostic and Statistical Manual of Mental Disorders*, Third Edition, Revised. Washington, DC: American Psychiatric Press.

American Society of Addiction Medicine (1991) *ASAM Patient Placement Criteria for the Treatment of Psychoactive Substance Use Disorders.* Washington, DC: American Society of Addiction Medicine, Inc.

Annis, H.M. & Davis, C.S. (1989) Relapse prevention. In *Handbook of Alcoholism Treatment Approaches: Effective Alternatives*, ed. Hester, R.K. & Miller, W.R. New York: Pergamon Press, 170–82.

Anton, R.F. & Moak, D.H. (1994) Carbohydrate deficient transferrin (CDT) and gamma-glutamyl transferase (GGT) as markers of heavy alcohol consumption: gender differences. *Alcoholism: Clinical and Experimental Research*, **18**, 653–6.

Ashton, M. (1999) Project MATCH: unseen colossus. *Drug and Alcohol Findings*, **1**, 15–21.

Babor, T.F. (1996) Reliability of the Ethanol Dependence Syndrome Scale. *Psychology of Addictive Behaviors*, **10**, 97–103.

Babor, T.F., Brown, J. & Del Boca, F.K. (1990) Validity of self-reports in applied research on addictive behaviors: fact or fiction? *Behavioral Assessment*, **12**, 5–31.

Babor, T.F., Cooney, N.L. & Lauerman, R.J. (1987a) The drug dependence syndrome concept as a psychological theory of relapse behaviour: an empirical evaluation of alcoholic and opiate addicts. *British Journal of Addiction*, **82**, 393–405.

Babor, T.F., Del Boca, F.K., McLaney, M.A., Jacobi, B., Higgins-Biddle, J. & Hass, W. (1991) Just say Y.E.S.: matching adolescents to appropriate interventions for alcohol and drug-related problems. *Alcohol Health and Research World*, **15**, 77–86.

Babor, T.F., Dolinsky, Z., Rounsaville, B.J. & Jaffe, J.H. (1989) Unitary versus multidimensional models of alcoholism treatment outcome: an empirical study. *Journal of Studies on Alcohol*, **49**, 167–77.

Babor, T.F., Hofmann, M., Del Boca, F.K. et al. (1992) Types of alcoholics. I: Evidence for an empirically derived typology based on indicators of vulnerability and severity. *Archives of General Psychiatry*, **49**, 599–608.

Babor T.F. & Lauerman, R.J. (1986) Classification and forms of inebriety: historical antecedents of alcoholic typologies. In *Recent Developments in Alcoholism*, Vol. 4, ed. Galanter, M. New York: Plenum Press, 113–44.

Babor T.F., Lauerman, R. & Cooney, N. (1987b) In search of the alcohol dependence syndrome: a cross national study of its structure and validity. In *Cultural Studies on Drinking and Drinking Problems*, ed. Paakkanen, P. & Sulkunen, P. Helsinki: Reports from the Social Research Institute of Alcohol Studies, 75–82.

Babor, T.F., Longabaugh, R., Zweben, A. et al. (1994) Issues in the definition and measurement of drinking outcomes in alcoholism treatment research. *Journal of Studies on Alcohol*, Suppl. 12, 101–11.

Babor, T.F., Steinberg, K., Anton, R. & Del Boca, F. (2000) Talk is cheap: measuring drinking outcomes in clinical trials. *Journal of Studies on Alcohol*, **61**, 55–63.

Bandura, A. (1986) *Social Foundations of Thought and Action: a Social Cognitive Theory*. Englewood Cliffs, NJ: Prentice-Hall.

Barrett, D. & Morse, P. (1998) Handling noncompliance. In *Strategies for Facilitating Protocol Compliance in Alcoholism Treatment Research*, Vol. 7, ed. Zweben, A., Barrett, D., Carty, K., McRee, B., Morse, P. & Rice, C. Project MATCH Monograph Series. Rockville, MD: National Institute of Alcohol Abuse and Alcoholism, 33–63.

Beattie, M.C., Longabaugh, R. & Fava, J. (1992) Assessment of alcohol-related workplace activities: development and testing of 'your workplace.' *Journal of Studies on Alcohol*, **53**, 469–75.

Beck, A.T., Steer, R.A. & Brown, G.K. (1986) *Beck Depression Inventory – Second Edition Manual*. San Antonio, TX: Psychological Corporation, Harcourt, Brace.

Beck, A.T., Ward, C.H., Mendelson, M., Mock, J. & Erbaugh, J. (1961) An inventory for measuring depression. *Archives of General Psychiatry*, **4**, 561–71.

Beckman, L.J. (1978) Self-esteem of women alcoholics. *Journal of Studies on Alcohol*, **39**, 491–8.

Bergin, A.E. & Garfield, S.L. (eds) (1994) *Handbook of Psychotherapy and Behavior Change*. New York: Wiley.

Beutler, L.E. (1991) Have all won and must all have prizes? Revisiting Luborsky et al.'s verdict. *Journal of Consulting and Clinical Psychology*, **59**, 226–32.

Beutler, L.E., Machado, P.O. & Neufeldt, S.A. (1994) Therapist variables. In *Handbook of Psychotherapy and Behavior Change*, ed. Bergin, A.E. & Garfield, S.L. New York: Wiley, 229–69.

Bien, T.H., Miller, W.R. & Tonigan, J.S. (1993) Brief interventions for alcohol problems: a review. *Addiction*, **88**, 315–35.

Blouin, A.G., Perez, E.L. & Blouin, J.H. (1988) Computerized administration of the Diagnostic Interview Schedule. *Psychiatric Research*, **23**, 335–44.

Bornstein, R.F. (1992) The dependent personality: developmental, social and clinical perspectives. *Psychological Bulletin*, **112**, 3–23.

Bryk, A.S. & Raudenbush, S.W. (1987) Application of hierarchical linear models to assessing change. *Psychological Bulletin*, **101**, 147–58.

Bufe, C. (1991) *Alcoholics Anonymous: Cult or Cure?* San Francisco: Sharp Press.

Caldwell, P.E. & Cutter, H.S.G. (1998) Alcoholics Anonymous affiliation during early recovery. *Journal of Substance Abuse Treatment*, **15**, 221–9.

Carbonari, J.P. & DiClemente, C.C. (2000) Using transtheoretical model profiles to differentiate levels of alcohol abstinence success. *Journal of Consulting and Clinical Psychology*, **68**, 810–17.

Carbonari, J.P., Wirtz, P.W., Muenz, L.R. & Stout, R.L. (1994) Alternative analytical methods for detecting matching effects in treatment outcomes. *Journal of Studies on Alcohol*, Suppl. 12, 83–90.

Carroll, K.M. (1996) Relapse prevention as a psychosocial treatment: a review of controlled trials. *Experimental and Clinical Pharmacology*, **4**, 46–54.

Carroll, K.M., Cooney, N.L., Donovan, D.M. et al. (1998) Internal validity of Project MATCH treatments: discriminability and integrity. *Journal of Consulting and Clinical Psychology*, **66**, 290–303.

Carroll, K.M., Kadden, R.M., Donovan, D.M., Zweben, A. & Rounsaville, B. (1994) Implementing treatment and protecting the validity of the independent variable in treatment matching studies. *Journal of Studies on Alcohol*, Suppl. 12, 149–55.

Chaney, E.F. (1989) Social skills training. In *Handbook of Alcoholism Treatment Approaches*, ed. Hester, R.K. & Miller, W.R. New York: Pergamon, 206–21.

Cisler, R., Holder, H.D., Longabaugh, R., Stout, R.L. & Zweben, A. (1998) Actual and estimated replication costs for alcohol treatment modalities: case study from Project MATCH. *Journal of Studies on Alcohol*, **59**, 503–12.

Cisler, R.A. & Zweben, A. (1999) Development of a composite measure for assessing alcohol treatment outcome: operationalization and validation. *Alcoholism: Clinical and Experimental Research*, **23**, 263–71.

Clifford, P.R. & Longabaugh, R. (1991) *Manual for the Administration of the Important People and Activities Instrument*. Providence, RI: Brown University Center for Alcohol and Addiction Studies.

Cohen, J. (1988) *Statistical Power Analysis for the Behavioral Sciences*, 2nd edn. Hillsdale, NJ: Lawrence Erlbaum.

Connors, G.J., Carroll, K.M., DiClemente, C.C., Longabaugh, R. & Donovan, D.M. (1997) The therapeutic alliance and its relationship to alcoholism treatment participation and outcome. *Journal of Consulting and Clinical Psychology*, **65**, 588–98.

Connors, G.J., DiClemente, C.C., Dermen, K.H., Kadden, R., Carroll, K.M. & Frone, M.R. (2000) Predicting the therapeutic alliance in alcoholism treatment. *Journal of Studies on Alcohol*, **61**, 139–49.

Connors, G.J., Tonigan, J.S. & Miller, W.R. (1996) A measure of religious background and behavior for use in behavior change research. *Psychology of Addictive Behaviors*, **10**, 90–6.

Connors, G.J., Tonigan, J.S. & Miller, W.R. (2001) Religiosity and responsiveness to alcoholism treatments: matching findings and causal chain analyses. In *Project MATCH Hypotheses: Results and Causal Chain Analyses*, Project MATCH Monograph Series, Vol. 8, NIH Publication No. 01-4238, ed. Longabaugh, R. & Wirtz, P. Bethesda, MD: National Institute on Alcohol Abuse and Alcoholism, 166–75.

Cook, C.H. (1988) Minnesota Model in the management of drug and alcohol dependency: miracle, method or myth? Part I. The philosophy and the programme. *British Journal of Addiction*, **83**, 625–34.

Cooney, N.L., Babor, T.F. & Litt, M.D. (2001). Matching clients to alcoholism treatment based on severity of alcohol dependence. In *Project MATCH Hypotheses: Results and Causal Chain Analyses*, Project MATCH Monograph Series, Vol. 8, NIH Publication No. 01-4238, ed. Longabaugh, R. & Wirtz, P. Bethesda, MD: National Institute on Alcohol Abuse and Alcoholism, 30–43.

Cooney, N.L., Kadden, R.M. & Litt, M.D. (1990) A comparison of methods for assessing sociopathy in male and female alcoholics. *Journal of Studies on Alcohol*, **51**, 42–8.

Cooney, N.L., Kadden, R.M., Litt, M.D. & Getter, H. (1991) Matching alcoholics to coping skills or interactional therapies: two year follow-up results. *Journal of Consulting and Clinical Psychology*, **59**, 598–601.

Cox, D.R. (1972) Regression models and life tables. *Journal of the Royal Statistical Society* (Series B), **34**, 187–220.

Crits-Christoph, P., Baranackie, K., Kurcias, J. et al. (1991) Meta-analysis of therapist effects in psychotherapy outcome studies. *Psychotherapy Research*, **1**, 81–91.

Crits-Christoph, P., Beebe, K.L. & Connolly, M.B. (1990) Therapist effects in the treatment of drug dependence: implications for conducting comparative treatment studies. In *Psychotherapy and Counseling in the Treatment of Drug Abuse*, ed. Onken, L.S. Rockville, MD: National Institute on Drug Abuse, 39–49.

Crumbaugh, J.C. (1977a) *The Seeking of Noetic Goals Test*. Murfreesboro, TN: Psychometric Affiliates.

Crumbaugh, J.C. (1977b) The Seeking of Noetic Goals Test (SONG): a complementary scale to the Purpose of Life Test (PLT). *Journal of Clinical Psychology*, **33**, 900–7.

Crumbaugh, J.C. & Maholick, L.T. (1976) *Purpose in Life Scale*. Murfreesboro, TN: Psychometric Affiliates.

Dance, K.A. & Neufeld, R.W.J. (1988) Aptitude-treatment interaction research in the clinical setting: a review of attempts to dispel the 'patient uniformity' myth. *Psychological Bulletin*, **104**, 192–213.

Deffenbacher, J.L., Thwaites, G.A., Wallace, T.L. & Oetting, E.R. (1994) Social skills and cognitive-relation approaches to general anger reduction. *Journal of Counseling Psychology*, **41**, 386–96.

Del Boca, F.K., Babor, T.F. & McRee, B. (1994) Reliability enhancement and estimation in multisite clinical trials. *Journal of Studies on Alcohol*, Suppl. 12, 130–6.

Del Boca, F.K. & Brown, J.M. (1996) Issues in the development of reliable measures in addictions research: introduction to Project MATCH assessment strategies. *Psychology of Addictive Behaviors*, **10**, 67–74.

Del Boca, F.K. & Noll, J.A. (2000) Truth or consequences: the validity of self-report data in health services research on addictions. *Addiction*, **95**, 347–60.

DiClemente, C.C. (1986) Self-efficacy and the addictive behaviors. *Journal of Social and Clinical Psychology*, **4**, 302–15.

DiClemente, C.C., Carbonari, J., Montgomery, R. & Hughes, S. (1994a) The Alcohol Abstinence Self-efficacy Scale. *Journal of Studies on Alcohol*, **55**, 141–8.

DiClemente, C.C., Carbonari, J.P. & Velasquez, M.M. (1992) Alcoholism treatment mismatching from a process of change perspective. In *Treatment of Drug and Alcohol Abuse*, ed. Watson, R.R. Totowa, NJ: Humana Press, 115–42.

DiClemente, C.C., Carbonari, J.P., Walker-Daniels, J., Donovan, D.M., Bellino, L.E. & Neavins, T.M. (2001a) Self-efficacy as a secondary matching hypothesis: causal chain analysis. In *Project MATCH Hypotheses: Results and Causal Chain Analyses*. Project MATCH Monograph Series, Vol. 8, NIH Publication No. 01-4238, ed. Longabaugh, R. & Wirtz, P. Bethesda, MD: National Institute on Alcohol Abuse and Alcoholism, 239–59.

DiClemente, C.C., Carbonari, J., Zweben, A., Morrel, T. & Lee, R.E. (2001b) Motivation hypothesis causal chain analysis. In *Project MATCH Hypotheses: Results and Causal Chain Analyses*. Project MATCH Monograph Series, Vol. 8, NIH Publication No. 01-4238, ed. Longabaugh, R. & Wirtz P. Bethesda, MD: National Institute on Alcohol Abuse and Alcoholism, 206–22.

DiClemente, C.C., Carroll, K.M., Connors, G.J. & Kadden, R.M. (1994b) Process assessment in treatment matching research. *Journal of Studies on Alcohol*, Suppl. 12, 156–62.

DiClemente, C.C. & Hughes, S.O. (1990) Stages of change profiles in outpatient alcoholism treatment. *Journal of Substance Abuse*, **2**, 217–35.

DiClemente, C.C. & Prochaska, J.O. (1998) Toward a comprehensive, trans-theoretical model of change: stages of change and addictive behaviors. In *Treating Addictive Behaviors*, 2nd edn, ed. Miller, W.R. & Heather, N. New York: Plenum Press, 3–24.

DiClemente, C.C. & Scott, C.W. (1997) Stages of change: interaction with treatment compliance and involvement. In *Beyond the Therapeutic Alliance: Keeping the Drug-dependent Individual in Treatment*, ed. Onken, L.S., Blaine, J.D. & Boren, J.J. Rockville, MD: National Institute on Drug Abuse, 131–56.

Dimeff, L.A. & Marlatt, G.A. (1998) Preventing relapse and maintaining change in addictive behaviors. *Clinical Psychology: Science and Practice*, **5**, 513–25.

Donovan, D.M. & Chaney, E.F. (1985) Alcoholic relapse: models and methods. In *Relapse Prevention: Maintenance Strategies in the Treatment of Addictive Behaviors*, ed. Marlatt, G. A. & Gordon, V. New York: Guilford Press, 351–416.

Donovan, D.M., Kadden, R.M., DiClemente, C.C. et al. (1994) Issues in the selection and development of therapies in alcoholism treatment matching research. *Journal of Studies on Alcohol*, Suppl. 12, 138–48.

Donovan, D.M., Kadden, R.M., DiClemente, C.C. & Carroll, K.M. (in press) Client satisfaction with three therapies in the treatment of alcohol dependence: results from Project MATCH. *American Journal on Addictions*.

Donovan, D., Kivlahan, D., Walker, R.D. & Umlauf, R. (1985) Derivation and validation of neuropsychological clusters among men alcoholics. *Journal of Studies on Alcohol*, 46, 205–11.

Donovan, D.M. & Marlatt, G.A. (1993) Behavioral treatment of alcoholism: a decade of evolution. In *Recent Developments in Alcoholism*, Vol. 11, ed. Galanter, M. New York: Plenum Press, 397–411.

Donovan. D.M. & Mattson, M.E. (1994) Alcoholism treatment matching research: methodological and clinical issues. *Journal of Studies on Alcoholism*, Suppl. 12, 5–14.

Duckert, F. (1987) Recruitment into treatment and effects of treatment for female problem drinkers. *Addictive Behaviors*, 12, 137–50.

Duckitt, A., Brown, D., Edwards, G., Oppenheimer, E., Sheehan, M. & Taylor, C. (1985) Alcoholism and the nature of outcome. *British Journal of Addiction*, 80, 153–62.

Edwards, G. (1986) The Alcohol Dependence Syndrome: usefulness of an idea. In *Alcoholism: New Knowledge and New Responses*, ed. Edwards, G. & Grant, M. London: Croom Helm, 136–56.

Edwards, G., Brown, D., Oppenheimer, E., Sheehan, M., Taylor, C. & Duckitt, A. (1988) Long term outcome for patients with drinking problems: the search for predictors. *British Journal of Addiction*, 83, 917–27.

Edwards, G. & Gross, M.M. (1976) Alcohol dependence: provisional description of a clinical syndrome. *British Medical Journal*, 1, 1058–61.

Edwards, G. & Taylor, C. (1994) A test of the matching hypothesis: alcohol dependence, intensity of treatment and 12-month outcome. *Addiction*, 89, 553–61.

Elkin, I., Parloff, M.B., Hadley, S.W. & Autry, J.H. (1985) NIMH treatment of depression collaborative research program: background and research plan. *Archives of General Psychiatry*, 42, 305–16.

Elkin, I., Shea, M.T., Watkins, J.T. et al. (1989) NIMH treatment of depression collaborative research program: general effectiveness of treatments. *Archives of General Psychiatry*, 46, 971–82.

Emrick, C.D. (1987) Alcoholics Anonymous: affiliation processes and effectiveness as treatment. *Alcoholism: Clinical and Experimental Research*, 11, 416–23.

Emrick, C.D. (1999) Alcoholics Anonymous and other 12 step groups. In *American Psychiatric Press Textbook of Substance Abuse Treatment*, 2nd edn, ed. Galanter, M. & Kleber, H.D. Washington, DC: The Press, 403–12.

Emrick, C.D. & Hansen, J. (1983) Assertations regarding effectiveness of treatment for alcoholism: fact or fantasy? *American Psychologist*, 38, 1078–88.

Emrick, C.D., Tonigan, J.S., Montgomery, H. & Little, L. (1993) Alcoholics Anonymous: what is currently known? In *Research on Alcoholics Anonymous:*

Opportunities and Alternatives, ed. McCrady, B.S. & Miller, W.R. New Brunswick, NJ: Rutgers Center of Alcohol Studies, 41–78.

Ewing, J.A. (1977) Matching therapy and patients: the cafeteria plan. *British Journal of Addiction*, **72**, 13–18.

Feragne, M.A., Longabaugh, R. & Stevenson, J.F. (1983) The Psychosocial Functioning Inventory. *Evaluation and Health Professionals*, **6**, 25–48.

Fichter, J.H. (1982) *The Rehabilitation of Clergy Alcoholics: Ardent Spirits Subdued.* New York: Human Sciences Press.

Finney, J.W. (1995) Enhancing substance abuse treatment evaluations: examining mediators and moderators of treatment effects. *Journal of Substance Abuse*, **7**, 135–50.

Finney, J.W. & Moos, R.J. (1986) Matching patients with treatments: conceptual and methodological issues. *Journal of Studies on Alcohol*, **7**, 122–34.

Finney, J.W., Moos, R.J. & Mewborn, C.R. (1980) Post-treatment experiences and treatment outcome of alcoholic patients six months and two years after hospitalization. *Journal of Consulting and Clinical Psychology*, **48**, 17–29.

Frank, J. (1976) *Persuasion and Healing: a Comparative Study of Psychotherapy.* Baltimore, MD: Johns Hopkins University Press.

Frosch, J.P. (1983) The treatment of antisocial and borderline personality disorders. *Hospital and Community Psychiatry*, **34**, 243–8.

Fuller, R.K., Mattson, M.E., Allen, J.P., Randall, C.L., Anton, R.F. &. Babor, T.F. (1994) Multisite clinical trials in alcoholism treatment research: organizational, methodological, and management issues. *Journal of Studies on Alcohol*, Suppl. 12, 30–7.

Galaif, E.R. & Sussman, S. (1995) For whom does Alcoholics Anonymous work? *International Journal of the Addictions*, **30**, 161–84.

Gallavardin, D. (1890) *The Homoeopathic Treatment of Alcoholism.* Philadelphia, PA: Hahnemann Publishing House.

Gartner, L. & Mee-Lee, D. (1995) *The Role of Current Status of Patient Placement Criteria in the Treatment of Substance Use Disorders.* Rockville, MD: US Department of Health and Human Services.

Gerstley, L., McLellan, A.T., Alterman, A.I., Woody, G.E., Luborsky, L. & Prout, M. (1989) Ability to form an alliance with the therapist: a possible marker of prognosis for patients with antisocial personality disorder. *American Journal of Psychiatry*, **146**, 508–12.

Glaser, F. (1980) Anybody got a match? Treatment research and the matching hypothesis. In *Alcoholism Treatment and Transition*, ed. Edwards, G. & Grant, M. London: Croom Helm, 178–96.

Glaser, F.B. & Skinner, H.A. (1981) Matching in the real world: a practical approach. In *Matching Patient Needs and Treatment Methods in Alcoholism and Drug Abuse*, ed. Gottheil, E., McLellan, A.T. & Druley, K.A. Springfield, IL: Charles C Thomas, 295–324.

Godlaski, T.M., Leukefeld, C. & Cloud, R. (1997) Recovery: with and without self-help. *Substance Use and Misuse*, **32**, 621–7.

Goldfried, M.R. (1980) Toward the delineation of therapeutic change principles. *American Psychologist*, **35**, 991–9.

Goodman, A.C., Holder, H.D., Nishiura, E. & Hankin, J.R. (1992) A discrete choice model of alcoholism treatment location. *Medical Care*, **30**, 1097–109.

Gottheil, E., Sterling, R.C., Weinstein, S.P. & Kurtz, J.W. (1994) Therapist/patient matching and early treatment dropout. *Journal of Addictive Diseases*, **13**, 169–76.

Gough, H.G. (1975) *California Psychological Inventory Manual*. Palo Alto, CA: Consulting Psychologists Press.

Gough, H.G. (1987) *California Psychological Inventory: Administrator's Guide*. Palo Alto, CA: Consulting Psychologists Press.

Hall, W., Saunders, J.B., Babor, T.F. et al. (1993) The structure and correlates of alcohol dependence: WHO collaborative project on the early detection of persons with harmful alcohol consumption III. *Addiction*, **88**, 1627–36.

Hartman, L., Krywonis, M. & Morrison, E. (1988) Psychological factors and health-related behavior change: preliminary findings from a controlled study. *Canadian Family Physician*, **34**, 1045–50.

Hasin, D.S. & Grant, B.F. (1995) AA and other help seeking for alcohol problems: former drinkers in the U.S. general population. *Journal of Substance Abuse*, **7**, 281–92.

Heather, N. (1989) Brief intervention strategies. In *Handbook of Alcoholism Treatment Approaches*, ed. Hester, R.K. & Miller, W.R. Elmsdorf, NY: Pergamon Press, 93–116.

Hesselbrock, M., Babor, T.F. Hesselbrock, V.R., Meyer E. & Workman, K. (1983) Never believe an alcoholic? On the validity of self-report measures of alcohol dependence and related constructs. *International Journal of the Addictions*, **18**, 593–609.

Hesselbrock, M., Hesselbrock, V., Babor, T., Stabenau, J., Meyer, R. & Weidenman, M. (1984) Antisocial behavior, psychopathology, and problem drinking in the natural history of alcoholism. In *Longitudinal Research in Alcoholism*, ed. Goodwin, I.D., Van Dusen, K. & Mednick, S.A. Norwell, MA: Kluwer Academic, 197–214.

Hester, R.K. & Miller, W.R. (eds) (1989) *Handbook of Alcoholism Treatment Approaches: Effective Alternatives*. New York: Pergamon Press.

Hester, R.K. & Miller, W.R. (eds) (1995) *Handbook of Alcoholism Treatment Approaches: Effective Alternatives*, 2nd edn. Boston, MA: Allyn & Bacon.

Hirschfeld, R.M., Klerman, G.L., Gough, G.H., Barrett, J., Korchin, S.J. & Chodoff, P. (1977) A measure of interpersonal dependency. *Journal of Personality Assessment*, **41**, 610–18.

Hoffmann, N.G. & Miller, N.S. (1992) Treatment outcomes for abstinence-based programs. *Psychiatric Annuals*, **22**, 402–8.

Holder, H., Longabaugh, R., Miller, W.R. & Rubonis, A.V. (1991) The cost effectiveness of treatment for alcoholism: a first approximation. *Journal of Studies on Alcohol*, **52**, 517–40.

Horn, J.L., Wanberg, K.W. & Foster, F.M. (1990) *Guide to the Alcohol Use Inventory*. Minneapolis, MN: National Computer Systems, Inc.

Horvath, A.O. & Greenberg, L. (1986) The development of the Working Alliance Inventory. In *The Psychotherapeutic Process: a Research Handbook*, ed. Greenberg, L.S. & Pinsof, W.M. New York: Guilford Press, 529–56.

Horvath, A.O. & Greenberg, L.S. (1994) *The Working Alliance: Theory, Research, and Practice.* New York: John Wiley.

Horvath, A.O. & Symonds B.D. (1991) Relation between working alliance and outcome and psychotherapy: a meta-analysis, *Journal of Counseling Psychology*, **38**, 139–49.

Horwitz, R.I., Viscoli, C.M., Clemens, J.D. & Sadock, R.T. (1990) Developing improved observational methods for evaluating therapeutic effectiveness. *American Journal of Medicine*, **89**, 630–8.

Hudson, H.L. (1985) How and why Alcoholics Anonymous works for blacks. *Alcoholism Treatment Quarterly*, **2**, 11–30.

Humphreys, K. (1997) Clinicians' referral and matching of substance abuse patients to self-help groups after treatment. *Psychiatric Services*, **48**, 1445–9.

Humphreys, K., Huebsch, P.D., Finney, J.W. & Moos, R.H. (1999) A comparative evaluation of substance abuse treatment: V. Substance abuse treatment can enhance the effectiveness of self-help groups. *Alcoholism: Clinical and Experimental Research*, **23**, **3**, 558–63.

Humphreys, K., Kaskutas, L.A. & Weisner, C. (1998) The Alcoholics Anonymous Affiliation Scale: development, reliability, and norms for diverse treated and untreated populations. *Alcoholism: Clinical and Experimental Research*, **22**, 974–8.

Humphreys, K., Mavis, B. & Stofflemayr, B. (1991) Factors predicting attendance at self-help groups after substance abuse treatment: preliminary findings. *Journal of Consulting and Clinical Psychology*, **59**, 591–3.

Humphreys, K. & Moos, R.H. (1996) Reduced substance-abuse-related health care costs among voluntary participants in Alcoholics Anonymous. *Psychiatric Services*, **47**, 709–13.

Hunt, D.E., Butler, L.F., Noy, L.E. & Rosser, M.E. (1978) *Assessing Conceptual Level by the Paragraph Completion Method.* Toronto: Ontario Institute for Studies in Education.

Institute of Medicine (1989) *Prevention and Treatment of Alcohol Problems: Research Opportunities.* Washington, DC: National Academy Press.

Institute of Medicine (1990) *Broadening the Base of Treatment for Alcohol Problems.* Washington, DC: National Academy Press.

Ito, J.R. & Donovan, D.M. (1986) Aftercare in alcoholism treatment: a review. In *The Addictive Behaviors: Process of Change*, ed. Miller, W.R. & Heather, N. New York: Plenum Press, 435–56.

Jaffe, A.J., Rounsaville, B., Chang, G., Schottenfeld, R.S., Meyer, R.E. & O'Malley S.S. (1996) Naltrexone, relapse prevention, and supportive therapy with alcoholics: an analysis of patient treatment matching. *Journal of Consulting and Clinical Psychology*, **64**, 1044–53.

Jarvis, T.J. (1992) Implications of gender for alcohol treatment research: a quantitative and qualitative review. *British Journal of Addiction*, **87**, 1249–61.

Jellinek, E.M. (1960) *The Disease Concept of Alcoholism.* New Brunswick, NJ: Hillhouse Press.

Kabela, E. & Kadden, R. (1997) Practical strategies for improving client compliance with treatment. In *Improving Compliance with Alcoholism Treatment*, Project MATCH Monograph Series, Vol. 6, NIH Publication No. 97-4143, ed.

Carroll, K.M. Bethesda, MD: National Institute on Alcohol Abuse and Alcoholism, 15–50).

Kadden, R., Carroll, K., Donovan, D. et al. (eds) (1992a) *Cognitive–Behavioral Coping Skills Therapy Manual: a Clinical Research Guide for Therapists Treating Individuals with Alcohol Abuse and Dependence*, Project MATCH Monograph Series, Vol. 3. NIH Publication No. (ADM) 94-3724, Rockville, MD: National Institute on Alcohol Abuse and Alcoholism.

Kadden, R.M., Cooney, N.L., Getter, H. & Litt, M.D. (1989) Matching alcoholics to coping skills or interactional therapies: posttreatment results. *Journal of Consulting and Clinical Psychology*, **57**, 698–704.

Kadden, R.M., Litt, M.D., Cooney, N.L. & Busher, D.A. (1992b) Relationship between role-play measures of coping skills and alcoholism treatment outcome. *Addictive Behaviors*, **17**, 425–37.

Kazdin, A.E. (1979) Nonspecific treatment factors in psychotherapy outcome research. *Journal of Consulting and Clinical Psychology*, **47**, 846–51.

Kazdin, A.E. & Bass, D. (1989) Power to detect differences between alternative treatments in comparative psychotherapy outcome research. *Journal of Consulting and Clinical Psychology*, **57**, 138–47.

Kiesler, D.J. (1966) Some myths of psychotherapy, research and the search for a paradigm. *Psychological Bulletin*, **65**, 110–36.

Kingree, J.B. (1997) Measuring Affiliation with 12-step groups. *Substance Use & Misuse*, **32**, 181–94.

Kissen, B., Platz, A. & Su, W.H. (1970) Social and psychological factors in the treatment of chronic alcoholism. *Journal of Psychiatric Research*, **8**, 13–27.

Kranzler, H.R. (2000) Pharmacotherapy of alcoholism: gaps in knowledge and opportunities for research. *Alcohol & Alcoholism*, **35**, 537–47.

Krupnick, J.L., Sotsky, S.M., Simmens, S. et al. (1996) The role of the therapeutic alliance in psychotherapy and pharmacotherapy outcome: findings in the National Institute of Mental Health Treatment of Depression Collaborative Research Program. *Journal of Consulting and Clinical Psychology*, **64**, 532–9.

Lambert, M.J. & Bergin, A.E. (1994) The effectiveness of psychotherapy. In *Handbook of Psychotherapy and Behavior Change*, 4th edn, ed. Bergin, A.E. & Garfield, S.L. New York: John Wiley & Sons, 143–89.

Leake, G.J. & King A.S. (1977) Effect of counselor expectations on alcoholic recovery. *Alcohol Health & Research World*, **11**, 16–22.

Lewis, C.E., Rice, J. & Helzer, J.E. (1983) Diagnostic interactions: alcoholism and antisocial personality. *The Journal of Nervous Mental Disease*, **171**, 105–13.

Lindström, L. (1992) *Managing Alcoholism: Matching Clients to Treatments*. Oxford: Oxford University Press.

Lipsey, M.W. (1990) *Design Sensitivity: Statistical Power for Experimental Research*. Newbury Park, CA: Sage Publications.

Litt, M.D., Babor, T.F., Del Boca, F.K., Kadden, R.M. & Cooney, N.L. (1992) Types of alcoholics II: application of an empirically derived typology to treatment matching. *Archives of General Psychiatry*, **49**, 609–14.

Longabaugh, R. & Beattie, M. (1985) The health service delivery system: optimizing its cost effectiveness for alcohol abusers. In *Future Directions in Alcohol*

Abuse Treatment Research, ed. McCrady, B.S., Noel, N.E. & Nirenberg, T.D. Rockville, MD: National Institute on Alcohol Abuse and Alcoholism, 104–36.

Longabaugh, R., Beattie, M., Noel, N., Stout, R. & Malloy, P. (1993) The effect of social investment on treatment outcome. *Journal of Studies on Alcohol*, **54**, 465–78.

Longabaugh, R., Rubin, A., Malloy, P., Beattie, M., Clifford, P. R. & Noel, N. (1994a) Drinking outcomes of alcohol abusers diagnosed as antisocial personality disorder. *Alcoholism: Clinical and Experimental Research*, **18**, 778–85.

Longabaugh, R. & Wirtz, P. (eds) (2001) *Project MATCH Hypotheses: Results and Causal Chain Analyses*. Project MATCH Monograph Series, Vol. 8, NIH Publication No. 01-4238. Bethesda, MD: National Institute on Alcohol Abuse and Alcoholism.

Longabaugh, R., Wirtz, P.W., DiClemente, C.C. & Litt, M. (1994b) Issues in the development of client–treatment matching hypotheses. *Journal of Studies on Alcohol*, Suppl. 12, 46–59.

Longabaugh, R., Wirtz, P.W., Zweben, A. & Stout, R.L. (1998) Network support for drinking, Alcoholics Anonymous and long-term matching effects. *Addiction*, **93**, 1313–33.

Luborsky, L., Barber, J.P., Siqueland, L., McLellan, A.T. & Woody, G. (1997) Establishing a therapeutic alliance with substance abusers. In *Beyond the Therapeutic Alliance: Keeping the Drug-dependent Individual in Treatment*, ed. Onken, L.S., Blaine, J.D. & Boren, J.J. Rockville, MD: US Department of Health and Human Services, 233–44.

Luborsky, L. & DeRubeis, R. (1984) The use of psychotherapy treatment manuals: a small revolution in psychotherapy research style. *Clinical Psychology Review*, **4**, 5–14.

Luborsky, L., McLellan, A.T., Woody, G.E., O'Brien, C.P. & Auerbach, A. (1985) Therapist success and its determinants. *Archives of General Psychiatry*, **42**, 602–11.

Luborsky, L., Singer, B. & Luborsky, L. (1975) Comparative studies of psychotherapy. *Archives of General Psychiatry*, **32**, 995–1008.

Lyons, J.P., Welte, J.W., Brown, J.W., Sokolow, L. & Hynes, G. (1982) Variation in alcoholism treatment orientation: differential impact upon specific subpopulations. *Alcoholism: Clinical and Experimental Research*, **6**, 333–43.

MacAndrew, C. (1965) The differentiation of male alcohol outpatients from non-alcoholic psychiatric outpatients by means of the MMPI. *Quarterly Journal of Studies on Alcohol*, **26**, 238–46.

Marlatt, G.A. & Gordon, J.R. (eds) (1985) *Relapse Prevention: Maintenance Strategies in the Treatment of Addictive Behaviors*. New York: Guilford Press.

Mattson, M.E. & Allen, J.P. (1991) Research on matching alcoholic patients to treatments: findings, issues, and implications. *Journal of Addictive Diseases*, **11**(2), 33–49.

Mattson, M.E., Allen, J.P., Longabaugh, R., Nickless, C.J., Connors, G.J. & Kadden, R.M. (1994) A chronological review of empirical studies matching alcoholic clients to treatment. *Journal of Studies on Alcohol*, Suppl. 12, 16–29.

Mattson, M.E., Del Boca, F.K., Carroll, K.M. et al. (1998) Patient compliance in

Project MATCH: session attendance, predictors, and relationship to outcome. *Alcoholism: Clinical and Experimental Research*, **22**, 1328–39.

McCrady, B.S., Epstein, E.E. & Hirsch, L.S. (1996) Issues in the implementation of a randomized clinical trial that includes Alcoholics Anonymous: studying AA-related behaviors during treatment. *Journal of Studies on Alcohol*, **57**, 604–12.

McCrady, B.S., Epstein, E.E. & Hirsch, L.S. (1999) Maintaining change after conjoint behavioral alcohol treatment for men: outcomes at six months. *Addiction*, **94**, 1381–96.

McCrady, B.S. & Smith, D.E. (1986) Implications of cognitive impairment for treatment of alcoholism. *Alcoholism: Clinical and Experimental Research*, **10**, 145–9.

McElrath, D. (1997) Minnesota Model. *Journal of Psychoactive Drugs*, **29**, 141–4.

McKay, J.R., Longabaugh, R., Beattie, M.C., Maisto, S.A. & Noel, N.E. (1993) Does adding cojoint therapy to individually focused alcoholism treatment lead to better family functioning? *Journal of Substance Abuse*, **5**, 45–59.

McLachlan, J.F.C. (1972) Benefit from group therapy as a function of patient/therapist match on conceptual level. *Psychotherapy: Theory, Research and Practice*, **9**, 317–23.

McLachlan, J.F. (1974) Therapy strategies, personality orientation and recovery from alcoholism. *Canadian Psychiatric Association Journal*, **19**, 25–30.

McLellan, A.T., Childress, A.R., Griffith, J. & Woody, G.E. (1984) The psychiatrically severe drug abuse patient: methadone maintenance or therapeutic community? *American Journal of Drug and Alcohol Abuse*, **10**, 77–95.

McLellan, A.T., Grant, G.R., Zanis, D., Randall, M., Brill, P. & O'Brien, C.P. (1997) Problem-service 'matching' in addiction treatment. *Archives of General Psychiatry*, **54**, 730–5.

McLellan, A.T., Kushner, H., Metzger, D. et al. (1992) The fifth edition of the Addiction Severity Index. *Journal of Substance Abuse Treatment*, **9**, 199–213.

McLellan, A.T., Luborsky, L., Woody, G.E. & O'Brien, C.P. (1980) An improved diagnostic evaluation instrument for substance abuse patients: the Addiction Severity Index. *Journal of Nervous and Mental Disease*, **168**, 26–33.

McLellan, A.T., Luborsky, L., Woody, G.E., O'Brien, C.P. & Kron, R. (1981) Are the addiction-related problems of substance abusers really related? *Journal of Nervous and Mental Disease*, **169**, 232–9.

McLellan, A.T., Woody, G.E., Luborsky, L. & Goehl, L. (1988) Is the counselor an 'active ingredient' in substance abuse rehabilitation? An examination of treatment success among four counselors. *Journal of Nervous and Mental Disease*, **176**, 423–30.

McLellan, A.T., Woody, G.E., Luborsky, L., O'Brien, C.P. & Druley, R.A. (1983) Increased effectiveness of substance abuse treatment: a prospective study of patient–treatment matching. *Journal of Nervous and Mental Disease*, **171**, 597–605.

McRee, B. (1998) The role of a coordinating center in facilitating research compliance in a multisite clinical trial. In *Strategies for Facilitating Protocol Compliance in Alcoholism Treatment Research*, Project MATCH Monograph Series, Vol. 7,

NIH Publication No. 98-4144, ed. Zweben, A., Barrett, D., Carty, K., McRee, B., Morse, P. & Rice, C. Bethesda, MD: National Institute on Alcohol Abuse and Alcoholism, 93–114.

Miller, N.S. & Hoffmann, N.G. (1995) Addictions treatment outcomes. *Alcoholism Treatment Quarterly*, **12**, 41–55.

Miller, W.R. (1985) Motivation for treatment: a review with special emphasis on alcoholism. *Psychological Bulletin*, **98**, 84–107.

Miller, W.R. (1989a) Increasing motivation for change. In *Handbook of Alcoholism Treatment Approaches: Effective Alternatives*, ed. Hester, R.K. & Miller, W.R. Elmsdorf, NY: Pergamon Press, 67–80.

Miller, W.R. (1989b) Matching individuals with interventions. In *Handbook of Alcoholism Treatment Approaches: Effective Alternatives*, ed. Hester, R.K. & Miller, W.R. New York: Pergamon Press, 261–71.

Miller, W.R. (1996) *Manual for Form 90: a Structured Assessment Interview for Drinking and Related Behaviors*, Project MATCH Monograph Series, Vol. 5, NIH Publication No. 96-4004. Bethesda, MD: National Institute on Alcohol Abuse and Alcoholism.

Miller, W.R., Benefield, R.G. & Tonigan, J.S. (1993) Enhancing motivation for change in problem drinking: a controlled comparison of two therapist styles. *Journal of Consulting and Clinical Psychology*, **61**, 455–61.

Miller, W.R., Brown, J.M., Simpson, T.L. et al. (1995a) What works? A methodological analysis of the alcohol treatment outcome literature. In *Handbook of Alcoholism Treatment Approaches: Effective Alternatives*, 2nd edn, ed. Hester, R.K. & Miller, W.R. Boston, MA: Allyn & Bacon, 12–44.

Miller, W.R. & Cooney, N.L. (1994) Designing studies to investigate client–treatment matching. *Journal of Studies on Alcohol*, Suppl. 12, 38–45.

Miller, W.R., Crawford, V.L. & Taylor, C.A. (1979) Significant others as corroborative sources for problem drinkers. *Addictive Behaviors*, **4**, 67–70.

Miller, W.R. & Del Boca, F.K. (1994) Measurement of drinking behavior using the Form 90 family of instruments. *Journal of Studies on Alcohol*, Suppl. 12, 112–18.

Miller W.R. & Heather, N. (1998) *Treating Addictive Behaviors*, 2nd edn. New York: Plenum Press.

Miller, W.R. & Hester, R.K. (1986a) Inpatient alcoholism treatment: who benefits? *American Psychologist*, **41**, 794–805.

Miller, W.R. & Hester, R.K. (1986b) Matching problem drinkers with optimal treatments. In *The Addictive Behaviors: Processes of Change*, ed. Miller, W.R. & Heather, N. New York: Plenum Press, 175–203.

Miller, W.R. & Marlatt, G.A. (1984) *Manual for the Comprehensive Drinker Profile*. Odessa, FL: Psychological Assessment Resources.

Miller, W.R. & Rollnick, S. (1991) *Motivational Interviewing: Preparing People to Change Addictive Behavior*. New York: Guilford Press.

Miller, W.R. & Tonigan, J.S. (1996) Assessing drinkers' motivation for change: the Stages of Change Readiness and Treatment Eagerness Scale (SOCRATES). *Psychology of Addictive Behaviors*, **10**, 81–9.

Miller, W.R., Tonigan, J.S. & Longabaugh, R. (1995b) *The Drinker Inventory of Consequences (DrInC): an Instrument for Assessing Adverse Consequences of*

Alcohol Abuse, Project MATCH Monograph Series, Vol. 4, NIH Publication No. 95-3911. Rockville, MD: National Institute on Alcohol Abuse and Alcoholism.

Miller, W.R., Walters, S.T. & Bennett, M.E. (2001) How effective is alcoholism treatment? *Journal of Studies on Alcohol*, **62**, 211–20.

Miller, W.R., Zweben, A., DiClemente, C.C. & Rychtarik, R.G. (1992) *Motivational-enhancement Therapy Manual: a Clinical Research Guide for Therapists Treating Individuals with Alcohol Abuse and Dependence*, Project MATCH Monograph Series, Vol. 2, NIH Publication No. 94-3723. Rockville, MD: National Institute on Alcohol Abuse and Alcoholism.

Monahan, S.C. & Finney, J.W. (1996) Explaining abstinence rates following treatment for alcohol abuse: a quantitative synthesis of patient, research design and treatment effects. *Addiction*, **91**, 787–805.

Montgomery, H.A., Miller, W.R. & Tonigan, J.S. (1995) Does Alcoholics Anonymous involvement predict treatment outcome? *Journal of Substance Abuse Treatment*, **12**, 241–6.

Monti, P.M., Abrams, D.B., Kadden, R.M. & Cooney, N.L. (1989) *Treating Alcohol Dependence: a Coping Skills Training Guide*. New York: Guilford Press.

Moos, R.H., Finney, J.W. & Cronkite, R.C. (1990) *Alcoholism Treatment: Context, Process, and Outcome*. New York: Oxford University Press.

Morgenstern, J., Kahler, C., Frey, R. & Labouvie, E. (1996) Modeling therapeutic responses to 12 step treatment: optimal responders, non-responders and partial responders. *Journal of Substance Abuse*, **8**, 45–59.

Morgenstern, J., Labouvie, E., McCrady, B.S., Kahler, C.W. & Frey, R.M. (1997) Affiliation with Alcoholics Anonymous after treatment: a study of its therapeutic effects and mechanisms of action. *Journal of Consulting and Clinical Psychology*, **65**, 768–77.

Morgenstern, J. & Longabaugh, R. (2000) Cognitive behavioral treatment for alcohol dependence: a review of mediating mechanisms and effectiveness. *Addiction*, **95**, 1475–90.

Najavits, L.M. & Weiss, R.D. (1994) Variations in therapist effectiveness in the treatment of patients with substance use disorders: an empirical review. *Addiction*, **89**, 679–88.

Nowinski, J. & Baker, S. (1992) *The Twelve-step Facilitation Handbook: a Systematic Approach to Early Recovery from Alcoholism and Addiction*. New York: Lexington Books.

Nowinski, J., Baker, S. & Carroll, K. (1992) *Twelve Step Facilitation Therapy Manual: a Clinical Research Guide for Therapists Treating Individuals with Alcohol Abuse and Dependence*, Project MATCH Monograph Series, Vol. 1, NIH Publication No. 94-3722. Rockville, MD: National Institute on Alcohol Abuse and Alcoholism.

Ogborne, A.C. & Glaser, F.B. (1981) Characteristics of affiliates of Alcoholics Anonymous: a review of the literature. *Journal of Studies on Alcohol*, **42**, 661–75.

Orford, J., Oppenheimer, E. & Edwards, G. (1976) Abstinence or control: the outcome for excessive drinkers two years after consultation. *Behaviour Research and Therapy*, **14**, 409–18.

Ouimette, P.C., Finney, J.W. & Moos, R.H. (1997) Twelve-step and cognitive behavioral treatment for substance abuse: a comparison of treatment effectiveness. *Journal of Consulting and Clinical Psychology*, **65**, 230–40.

Ouimette, P.C., Finney, J.W., Gima, K. & Moos, R.H. (1999) A comparative evaluation of substance abuse treatment: examining mechanisms underlying patient–treatment matching hypotheses for 12-step and cognitive–behavioral treatments for substance abuse. *Alcoholism: Clinical and Experimental Research*, **23**, 545–51.

Ouimette P.C., Moos, R.H. & Finney, J.W. (1998) Influence of outpatient treatment and 12-step group involvement on one-year substance abuse treatment outcomes. *Journal of Studies on Alcohol*, **59**, 513–22.

Parsons, O.A. (1986) Alcoholics' neuropsychological impairment: current findings and conclusions. *Annals of Behavioral Medicine*, **8**, 13–19.

Patterson, G.R. & Forgatch, M.S. (1985) Therapist behavior as a determinant for client noncompliance: a paradox for the behavior modifier. *Journal of Consulting and Clinical Psychology*, **53**, 846–51.

Pattison, E.M., Sobell, M.B. & Sobell, L.C. (1977) *Emerging Concepts of Alcohol Dependence*. New York: Springer.

Pedhuaser, E.J. (1982) *Multiple Regression in Behavioral Research: Explanation and Prediction*, 2nd edn. New York: Holt, Rinehart, and Winston.

Pettinati, H.M., Meyers, K., Jenson, J.M., Kaplan, F. & Evans, B.D. (1993) Inpatient versus outpatient treatment for substance dependence revisited. *Psychiatric Quarterly*, **64**, 173–82.

Prochaska, J.O. & DiClemente, C.C. (1984) *The Transtheoretical Approach: Crossing the Traditional Boundaries of Therapy*. Malabar, FL: Krieger.

Prochaska, J.O. & DiClemente, C.C. (1992) Stages of change in the modification of problem behaviors. In *Progress in Behavior Modification*, Vol. 28, ed. Hersen, M., Eisler, R.M. & Miller, P.M. Sycamore, IL: Sycamore Publishing Company, 183–218.

Prochaska, J.O., DiClemente, C.C. & Norcross, J.C. (1992) In search of how people change: applications to addictive behaviors. *American Psychologist*, **47**, 1102–14.

Procidano, M.E. & Heller, K. (1983) Measures of perceived social support from friends and family: three validation studies. *American Journal of Community Psychology*, **11**, 1–24.

Project MATCH Research Group (1993) Project MATCH: rationale and methods for a multisite clinical trial matching patients to alcoholism treatment. *Alcoholism: Clinical and Experimental Research*, **17**, 1130–45.

Project MATCH Research Group (1997a) Matching alcoholism treatments to client heterogeneity: Project MATCH posttreatment drinking outcomes. *Journal of Studies on Alcohol*, **58**, 7–29.

Project MATCH Research Group (1997b) Project MATCH secondary a priori hypotheses. *Addiction*, **92**, 1671–98.

Project MATCH Research Group (1998a) Matching alcoholism treatments to client heterogeneity: Project MATCH three year drinking outcomes. *Alcoholism: Clinical and Experimental Research*, **22**, 1300–11.

Project MATCH Research Group (1998b) Matching alcoholism treatments to client heterogeneity: treatment main effects and matching effects on drinking during treatment. *Journal of Studies on Alcohol*, **59**, 631–9.

Project MATCH Research Group (1998c) Matching patients with alcohol disorders to treatments: clinical implications from Project MATCH. *Journal of Mental Health*, **7**, 589–602.

Project MATCH Research Group (1998d) Therapist effects in three treatments for alcohol problems. *Psychotherapy Research*, **8**, 455–74.

Regier, D.A., Farmer, M.E., Rae, D.S. et al. (1990). Comorbidity of mental disorders with alcohol and other drug abuse. *Journal of the American Medical Association*, **264**, 2511–18.

Reitan, R.M. (1958) Validity of the Trail Making Test as an indicator of organic brain damage. *Perceptual and Motor Skills*, **8**, 271–6.

Rice, C. & Longabaugh, R. (1996) Measuring general social support in alcoholic patients: short forms for perceived social support. *Psychology of Addictive Behaviors*, **10**, 104–14.

Robins, L., Helzer, J., Cottler, L. & Goldring, E. (1989) *NIMH Diagnostic Interview Schedule: Version III Revised (DIS-III-R), Question by Question Specifications*. St Louis, MO: Washington University.

Robins, L.N., Helzer, J.E., Croughan, J. & Ratcliff, K.S. (1981) National Institute of Mental Health Diagnostic Interview Schedule: its history, characteristics and validity. *Archives of General Psychiatry*, **38**, 381–9.

Rogers, C.R. (1957) The necessary and sufficient conditions of therapeutic personality change. *Journal of Consulting Psychology*, **21**, 95–103.

Rohsenow, D.J., Monti, P.M., Bindoff, J.A., Leipman, M.R., Nirenberg, T.D. & Abrams, D.B. (1991) Patient–treatment matching for alcoholic men in communication skills versus cognitive–behavioral mood management training. *Addictive Behaviors*, **16**, 63–9.

Room, R. (1993) Alcoholics Anonymous as a social movement. In *Research on Alcoholics Anonymous: Opportunities and Alternatives*, ed. McCrady, B.S. & Miller, W.R. New Brunswick, NJ: Rutgers Center of Alcohol Studies, 167–88.

Rounsaville, B.J., Dolinsky, Z.S., Babor, T.F. & Meyer, R.E. (1987) Psychopathology as a predictor of treatment outcome in alcoholics. *Archives of General Psychiatry*, **44**, 505–13.

SAS Institute (1992) *SAS Technical Report P-229*. Cary, NC: SAS Insitute.

Schwarz, N. (1999) Self-reports: how the questions shape the answers. *American Psychologist*, **54**, 93–105.

Shipley, W.C. (1940) A self-administered scale for measuring intellectual impairment and deterioration. *Journal of Psychology*, **9**, 371–7.

Shipley, W.C. (1946) *Shipley-Institute of Living Scale: Manual of Directions and Scoring Key*. Hartford, CT: Institute of Living.

Simpson, D.D, Joe, G.W., Rowan-Szal, G. & Greener, J. (1995) Client engagement in change during drug abuse treatment. *Journal of Substance Abuse*, **7**, 117–34.

Sisson, R.W. & Mallams, J.H. (1981) The use of systematic encouragement and community access procedures to increase attendance at Alcoholics Anonymous and Al-Anon meetings. *American Journal of Drug and Alcohol Abuse*, **8**, 371–6.

Skinner, H.A. (1981) Different strokes for different folks. Differential treatment for alcohol abuse. In *Evaluation of the Alcoholic: Implications for Research, Theory and Treatment*, ed. Meyer, R.E., Babor, T.F., Glueck, B.C., Jaffe, J., O'Brien, J. & Stabenan, J. Washington, DC: National Institute on Alcohol Abuse and Alcoholism, 349–67.

Sloane, R.B., Staples, F.R., Cristol, A.H., Yorkston, N.J. & Whipple, K. (1975) *Psychotherapy Versus Behavior Therapy*. Cambridge, MA: Harvard University Press.

Smith, A. (1973) *Symbol Digit Modalities Test*. Los Angeles, CA: Western Psychological Services.

Smith, B. & Sechrest, L. (1991) Treatment of aptitude by treatment interactions. *Journal of Consulting and Clinical Psychology*, **59**, 233–44.

Smith, K.J., Subich, L.M. & Kalodner, C. (1995) The transtheoretical model's stages and processes of change and their relation to premature termination. *Journal of Counseling Psychology*, **42**, 34–9.

Snow, M.G., Prochaska, J.O. & Rossi, J.S. (1994) Processes of change in Alcoholics Anonymous: maintenance factors in long-term sobriety. *Journal of Studies on Alcohol*, **55**, 362–71.

Snow, R.E. (1991) Aptitude-treatment interaction as a framework for research on individual differences in psychotherapy. *Journal of Consulting and Clinical Psychology*, **59**, 205–16.

Snyder, S.H. (1980) *Biological Aspects of Mental Disorders*. New York: Oxford University Press.

Sobell, L.C., Cunningham, J.A. & Sobell, M.B. (1996) Recovery from alcohol problems with and without treatment: prevalence in two population surveys. *American Journal of Public Health*, **86**, 966–72.

Sobell, L.C. & Sobell, M.B. (1992) Timeline follow-back: a technique for assessing self-reported alcohol consumption. In *Measuring Alcohol Consumption: Psychosocial and Biochemical Methods*, ed. Litten, R.Z. & Allen, J.P. Totowa, NJ: Humana Press, 41–72.

Sobell, M.B. & Sobell, L.C. (1998) Guiding self-change. In *Treating Addictive Behaviors*, 2nd edn, ed. Miller, W.R. & Heather, N. New York: Plenum Press, 189–202.

Sotsky, S.M., Glass, D.R., Shea, M.T. et al. (1991) Patient predictors of response to psychotherapy and pharmacotherapy: findings in the NIMH treatment of depression collaborative research program. *American Journal of Psychiatry*, **148**, 997–1008.

Spence, J.T., Helmreich, R. & Stapp, J. (1974) The Personal Attributes Questionnaire: a measure of sex role stereotypes and masculinity–femininity. *Catalog of Selected Documents in Psychology*, **4**, 43–4.

Spicer, J. (1993) *Minnesota Model: the Evolution of the Multidisciplinary Approach to Addiction Recovery*. Center City, MN: Hazelden Educational Materials.

Spielberger, C.D. (1988) *Manual for the State–Trait Anger Expression Scale (STAX)*. Odessa, FL: Psychological Assessment Resources, Inc.

Spielberger, C.D., Jacobs, G., Russel, S. & Crane, R.S. (1983) Assessment of anger: the state–trait anger scale. In *Advances in Personality Assessment*, Vol. 2, ed.

Butcher, J.N. & Spielberger, C.D. Hillsdale, NJ: Lawrence Erlbaum, 159–87.

Spitzer, R.L. & Williams, J.B.W. (1985) *Structured Clinical Interview for DSM-III-R, Patient Version*. New York: New York State Psychiatric Institute.

Sterling, R.C., Gottheil, E., Weinstein, S.P. & Serota, R. (1998) Therapist/patient race and sex matching: treatment retention and 9-month follow-up outcome. *Addiction*, **93**, 1043–50.

Stinchfield, R., Owen, P.L. & Winters, K.C. (1994) Group therapy for substance abuse: a review of the empirical literature. In *Handbook of Group Psychotherapy: an Empirical and Clinical Synthesis*, ed. Fuhriman, A. & Burlingame, G.M. New York: John Wiley & Sons, 458–88.

Stout, R.L., Wirtz, P.W., Carbonari, J.P. & Del Boca, F.K. (1994) Ensuring balanced distribution of prognostic factors in treatment outcome research. *Journal of Studies on Alcohol*, Suppl. 12, 70–5.

Tarter, R.E. (1983) The causes of alcoholism: a biopsychological analysis. In *Etiologic Aspects of Alcohol and Drug Abuse*, ed. Gottheil, E., Druley, K.A., Skoloda, T.E. & Waxman, H.M. Springfield, IL: Charles C Thomas, 173–201.

Tellegen, A. (1982) *Brief Manual for the Differential Personality Questionnaire*. Minneapolis, MN: University of Minnesota.

Timko, C., Finney, J.W., Moos, R.H. & Moos, B.S. (1995) Short-term treatment careers and outcomes of previously untreated alcoholics. *Journal of Studies on Alcohol*, **56**, 597–610.

Timko, C., Finney, J.W., Moos, R.H., Moos, B.S. & Steinbaum, D.P. (1993) The process of treatment selection among previously untreated help-seeking problem drinkers. *Journal of Substance Abuse*, **5**, 203–20.

Tonigan, J.S., Connors, G.J. & Miller, W.R. (1996a) The Alcoholics Anonymous Involvement (AAI) Scale: reliability and norms. *Psychology of Addictive Behaviors*, **10**, 75–80.

Tonigan, J.S. & Hiller-Sturmhofel, S. (1994) Alcoholics Anonymous: who benefits? *Alcohol Health and Research World*, **18**, 308–10.

Tonigan, J.S., Miller, W.R. & Brown, J.M. (1997) The reliability of Form 90: an instrument for assessing alcohol treatment outcome. *Journal of Studies on Alcohol*, **58**, 358–64.

Tonigan, J.S., Miller, W.R. & Connors, G.J. (2001) Prior Alcoholics Anonymous involvement and treatment outcome: matching findings and causal chain analyses. In *Project MATCH Hypotheses: Results and Causal Chain Analyses*, Project MATCH Monograph Series, Vol. 8, NIH Publication No. 01-4238, ed. Longabaugh, R. & Wirtz, P. Bethesda, MD: National Institute on Alcohol Abuse and Alcoholism, 276–84.

Tonigan, J.S., Toscova, R. & Miller, W.R. (1996b) Meta-analysis of the literature on Alcoholics Anonymous: sample and study of characteristics moderate findings. *Journal of Studies on Alcohol*, **57**, 65–72.

Truax, C.B. & Carkuff, R.R. (1967) *Toward Effective Counseling and Psychotherapy*. Chicago, IL: Alding.

Tuchfield, B. (1981) Spontaneous remission in alcoholics: empirical observations and theoretical implications. *Journal of Studies on Alcohol*, **42**, 626–41.

Valliant, G.E. (1995) *The National History of Alcoholism Revisited*. Cambridge, MA: Harvard University Press.

Velasquez, M.M., DiClemente, C.C. & Addy, R. (2000). The generalizability of Project MATCH: a comparison of clients enrolled to those not enrolled in the study at one aftercare site. *Drug and Alcohol Dependence*, **59**(2), 177–82.

Waldron, H., Miller, W.R. & Tonigan, J.S. (2001) Client Anger as a predictor to treatment response. In *Project MATCH: A Priori Matching Hypotheses, Results, and Mediating Mechanisms*, Project MATCH Monograph Series, Vol. 8, ed. Longabaugh, R.H. & Wirtz, P.W. Bethesda, MD: National Institute on Alcohol Abuse and Alcoholism, 134–48.

Walsh, D.C., Hingson, R.W., Merrigan, D.M. et al. (1991) A randomized trial of treatment options for alcohol-abusing workers. *New England Journal of Medicine*, **325**, 775–82.

Wanberg, K.W., Horn, J.L. & Foster, F.M. (1977) A differential assessment model for alcoholism: the scales of the Alcohol Use Inventory. *Journal of Studies on Alcohol*, **38**, 512–43.

Waskow, I.E. (1984) Specification of the technique variable in the NIMH treatment of depression collaborative research program. In *Psychotherapy Research: Where We Are and Where We Should Go*, ed. Williams, J.B.W. & Spitzer, R.L. New York: Guilford Press, 150–9.

Watson, C.G., Hancock, M., Gearhart, L.P., Mendez, C.M., Malovrh, P. & Raden, M. (1997) Comparative outcome study of frequent, moderate, occasional, and nonattenders of Alcoholics Anonymous. *Journal of Clinical Psychology*, **53**, 209–14.

Weissman, M.M., Rounsaville, B.J. & Chevron, E. (1982) Training psychotherapists to participate in psychotherapy outcome studies. *American Journal of Psychiatry*, **139**, 1442–6.

Welte, J., Hynes, G., Sokolow, L. & Lyons, J.P. (1981) Effect of length of stay in inpatient alcoholism treatment on outcome. *Journal of Studies on Alcohol*, **42**, 483–91.

White, W.L. (1998) *Slaying the Dragon. The History of Addiction Treatment and Recovery in America*. Bloomington, IL: Chestnut Health Systems.

Wirtz, P.W., Carbonari, J.P., Muenz, L.R., Stout, R.L., Tonigan, J.S. & Connors, G.J. (1994) Classical analytical methods for detecting matching effects on treatment outcome. *Journal of Studies on Alcohol*, Suppl. 12, 76–82.

Woody, G.E., McLellan, A.T., Luborsky, L. et al. (1984) Severity of psychiatric symptoms as a predictor of benefits from psychotherapy: the Veterans Administration. *American Journal of Psychiatry*, **141**, 1172–7.

Zweben, A., Barrett, D., Carty, K., McRee, B., Morse, P. & Rice, C. (eds) (1998) *Strategies for Facilitating Compliance in Alcoholism Treatment*, Project MATCH Monograph Series, Vol. 7, NIH Publication No. 98-4144. Bethesda, MD: National Institute on Alcohol Abuse and Alcoholism.

Zweben, A. & Cisler, R. (1996) Composite outcome measures in alcoholism treatment research: problems and potentialities. *Substance Use and Misuse*, **31**, 1783–805.

Zweben, A., Donovan, D.M., Randall, C.L. et al. (1994) Issues in the development of subject recruitment strategies and eligibility criteria in multisite trials of matching. *Journal of Studies on Alcohol*, Suppl. 12, 62–99.

Index

Note. Page numbers in *italics* refer to figures and tables. Alcoholics Anonymous is abbreviated to AA in subentries.

abstinence
  AA attendance   184–5, 199–202, 217, 231
  AA program   184–5
  client–treatment matching   213
  emphasizing in Twelve Step Facilitation (TSF)   146
  illicit drugs   152, 157
  intentional behavioral change   177, 180
  Outpatient arm   225
  prognostic indicators   215
  Project MATCH   220
  support   231
  treatment evaluation   151, 157, 210
  Twelve Step Facilitation   163, 220
  see also Percent Days Abstinent (PDA)
Addiction Severity Index (ASI)   31
  Psychiatric Severity measure   99
    Aftercare arm   138
    Outpatient arm   122, *123*, 124
    score   70, 93
    treatment effectiveness   133–4, 153
aftercare
  adjunct to outcome   21
  sites   18
Aftercare arm   135–49
  AA attendance   190–2, 193–4, 217
    alcohol dependence   227
    treatment evaluation   196
  AA prior engagement   145, 149
  AA utilization pattern   197–9
  alcohol and drug use   157
  alcohol dependence   143, *145*, 148–9, 223, 227
  hypothesis   146–7, 148–9
  ambulatory interventions   81
  causal chain analysis   146–7

client participation   25, *26*, 27
client–treatment matching   212
clinical deterioration   59
clinical trial   20–1
completion rates   138–9
composite outcome measures   154, *155*, *156*, 157
counseling   105
deaths   59
differences from Outpatient arm   225–7
exploratory analyses   145–6
follow-up   73, *74*, 75, 140–1
improvement levels   147
inclusion criteria   30
matching effects   147–9
outcome measures
  primary   164
  secondary   158, *159*
participant enrollment   63, *64*, 65
participants
  phase of life   164
  selection factors   164–5
prior treatment   148
prognostic effects   142, 215–16, 228
recruitment   226
  sites   136–7
research
  design   *26*
  participants   137–8
self-efficacy   180
sites   217–18
time to first drink   154, *156*
treatment choice   224
treatment manual   51
treatment outcomes   218, 226
trends over time   139, *140*, *141*
Working Alliance Inventory   174–5

Alcohol Abstinence Self-Efficacy (AASE)
  scale, Confidence subscale   101
alcohol abuse diagnosis   29–30
alcohol consumption
  baseline   40
  measurement   32
  recent   39
  see also drinking
alcohol dependence   96–7
  AA meeting attendance outcome   227
  Aftercare arm   143, *145*, 148–9, 223
  diagnosis   29–30
  motivation correlation   178
  prognostic indicator   215
  severity   21
  syndrome   96
alcohol dependence hypothesis
  AA involvement   146–7
  Aftercare arm   146–7, 148–9
alcohol involvement
  hypothesis   96
  matching hypotheses   85
  measures   35
  prognostic indicator   215
alcohol problem severity   220
alcohol-related consequences   160, *162*
alcohol-related problems, severity
        indicators   116–17
Alcohol Use Disorders Identification Test
        (AUDIT)   66
Alcohol Use Inventory (AUI)   31, 39
  alcohol involvement   85
  subscales   126–8
alcoholic typology index   31
alcoholics, recovering   229
Alcoholics Anonymous (AA)   184–5
  abstinence   184–5, 199–202, 217, 231
  Aftercare arm   190–2
  attendance at meetings   48, 54–5, 185,
        186
    abstinence   199, 201–2
    alcohol use   199–202
  benefits   204
  Form-90   188–9
  frequency   202
  initiation during treatment   203
  multivariate analysis   195
  outcome   227–8
  post-treatment   197–9
  predictors   146–7
  Project MATCH   187
  during treatment   149, 197–9
  treatment group differences   192–5
  commitment   23, 185
    Project MATCH   187
  confrontational style   91

dependency needs   98
disaffiliation   202–3
gender   91
involvement   186, 217
  measurement   70, 189–90
  outcome   91
  Outpatient arm   190–2
  patterns of utilization   196–9
  practice of related activities   202
  prior engagement   99, 145, 149
    motivation correlation   178
    prognostic effect   215
  reliability of measures   188–90
  sobriety goal   185
  subjective ratings   190
  treatability of alcoholism   4
  treatment evaluation   195–6
  Twelve Steps   23, 47, 169, 171, 184
    condition   187, 231
    involvement enhancement   227–8
    multifaceted orientation   186
  validity of measures   188–90
Alcoholics Anonymous Involvement scale
        99
alcoholism
  definitions   5
  etiology   95
  heterogeneity   5
  interventions   3–4, 13, 81
  recovery   133
  treatability   4
  Type A   95, 96
  Type B   95, 96
  typology   95–6
Ambivalence   100
American Society of Addiction Medicine
        Patient Placement Criteria   10
anger   97
  causal chain analysis   130
  client–treatment matching   212
  clinical significance   130
  hypothesis   130
  Motivational Enhancement Therapy   97,
        120, 124, 212, 219, 231
  sociopathy   94
  treatment outcome   *120*, 124, 126, 132
antisocial behavior, prognostic value   216
antisocial personality disorder   12, 97–8
  Aftercare arm   143, *144*, 145
  outcome   *120*, 122
anxiety
  concurrent   8
  levels   12
appointment flexibility   72
aptitude–treatment interaction (ATI)   11
a priori hypothesis tests   111, 143

assessment battery development 30–1
assessment sessions 33
audit, independent random 70–1

Beck Depression Inventory 153
behavioral change
    client role 181
    commitment 46
    dimensions 169
    engagement indicators 181
    experiential 179
    intentional 168–9, 177–81
    motivation 39, 45, 92
        intentional 177–9
        internal 23
    process 166–9, 179
    see also readiness to change
belief 234
best practice 228–30
Bonferroni correction 83, 109, 143

California Personality Inventory (CPI) 31
California Psychological Inventory,
    Socialization scale 94
carbohydrate-deficient transferrin (CDT)
    32, 35
causal chain analysis 128–9, 133, 231
    Aftercare arm 146–7
    matching hypotheses 213–14
causal chains 83
centralized urn randomization procedure
    67
certification protocol 69
change
    creation 234
    stage construct 92
    see also behavioral change
client characteristics 62, 63, 64, 65–6, 209
    assessment 169
    database 67
    personal problems 72
    prognostic indicators 216
    treatment outcomes 215–16
clients *see* participants
client–treatment interactions 13
client–treatment matching 21, 211–14
clinical assessment 29–41
    biological 32, 39
    data accuracy 40–1
    deterioration guidelines 58–9
    instruments
        administration 38–41
        selection 33–4
    methodology 38–9
    outcome effects 40
    practical considerations 40–1

sensitivity to recent alcohol consumption
    39
sessions 33
timing 39
Clinical Care Committee, clinical
    deterioration criteria 58–9
clinical judgment 8
Clinical Research Units (CRUs) 17,
    18–19, 238–9
    AA attendance 193
    Aftercare arm 136–7, 138, 139–40,
        147–8
    communication 20
    compliance monitoring 72
    consistency of interventions 51
    data input 70
    exploratory analyses 126
    Outpatient arm 106–7
    site effect covariates 110
    site visits 69
    treatment effects 115–16
    trends over time 115
clinical trials 3
    randomized 11, 22, 67, 236
clinical trials, multisite 15–28
    Aftercare arm 20–1
    challenges 16–17
    client participation 25, 26, 27
    clinical assessment 29–41
    communication 20
    control group absence 23–4
    data collection phase 69
    design 20–5, 26, 27
    exclusion criteria 29, 30
    follow-up evaluations 25
    inclusion criteria 29–30
    matching strategy 22
    matching variables 31
    measurement reliability 69–70
    Outpatient arm 20–1
    patient characteristic range 21
    process assessment 38
    prognostic variables 30–1
    project management 19
    random assignment 22
    rationale 16–17
    responsibility for planning/conducting
        17
    therapy implementation 56–7, 58
    treatment content 23
    treatment selection 22–3
cognitive impairment
    matching hypotheses 85, 90
    measurement 31, 90
    outcome 90
cognitive–behavioral approaches 12

Cognitive–Behavioral Therapy (CBT) 23, 43–5, *123*, 124
  AA attendance 192–5
    frequency 202
  alcohol dependence 96, 97, 147
  anger 97, *120*, 124
  behavioral change 92
  choice of therapy 224
  client satisfaction with treatment 176
  clinical deterioration 59
  clinical methods 44
  compliance 54
    outcome association 78
  costs 59–61
  crisis strategies 58
  exploratory analyses 127–8
  gender 91
  interpersonal dependency 98
  meaning seeking 143
  motivation time effect *120*, 122
  outcome 211
  psychiatric severity 93
    hypothesis matching 129
  psychopathology 99
  readiness to change 100, 145
  sessions 44–5
  social functioning 101
  sociopathy outcome 93–4
  Support for Drinking hypothesis 130–1
  techniques 169, *170*, 171
  therapeutic dimensions *56–7*
  therapists 45, 52, 171–2
  treatment
    client satisfaction 176
    effectiveness 219
    effects 115
    matching 223
  treatment manual 50–1
  trends over time 139, *140*, *141*
  typology of alcoholism 95
communication
  roles/responsibilities 71
  skills training 12
compliance 53–4, 73
  difficulties 73
  enhancement strategies 71–3
  levels of study 79
  monitoring 72
  treatment outcome association 77–80
Computerized Diagnostic Interview Schedule (C-DIS) 98, 99
conjoint couples therapy 12–13
control group absence 23–4, 182–3
Coordinating Center (CC) 17, 18, 20, 239
  compliance monitoring 72
  therapist training review 52–3

coping skills approaches 12, 43
counseling, outpatient 105
covariate analysis 109–10
data
  accuracy 75, *76*, 77
  audit 70–1
  completeness 73, *74*, 75
  missing 111–12
  processing/management 70–1
  quality indicators 73, 79
  timeliness 75
Data Safety and Monitoring Board (DSMB) 17–18
day-hospital treatment, intensive 18
dependence on other drugs 8
depression
  alcohol consumption relationship 160, *162*
  concurrent 8
  measurement 153
detoxification need 8
Diagnostic and Statistical Manual 29–30
  see also DSM *entries*
Drinker Inventory of Consequences 34, 39, 153
drinking
  age at onset 46
  assessment following treatment 152–3
  behavior assessment 152, 154, *155–6*, 157
  biological indicators 32, 39
  feedback on behavior 46
  frequency prediction 181
  functional relationship to coping 43–4
  heavy 152–3, 157
  negative consequences 32
  outcome assessment 169
  outcome variables 70
  post-treatment 159–60, *161–2*, 163, 164
  predictive value 163
  see also alcohol consumption
Drinks per Drinking Day (DDD) 32, 35, 107
  AA attendance 200, 201
  Aftercare arm 138, 139, *141*
  client satisfaction with treatment 177
  exploratory analyses 126
  follow-up analysis 112, 140
  secondary outcome correlation 160, *161*
  self-efficacy 180
  treatment effects 115, 116
  trends over time 114–15
drug use, illicit 65

abstinence 152, 157
alcohol consumption relationship 160, *162*
dependence 8
DSM-III-R
psychopathology diagnosis 99
sociopathy diagnosis 98
DSM-IV Structured Clinical Interview 69
DSM-R-III
alcohol dependence criteria 137–8
diagnosis of alcohol-use disorders 70

emergency sessions 58
environment, cognitive style of relating to 90–1
Ethanol Dependence Syndrome scale 70, 97
ethnic minorities, representation in project 66
exploratory data analysis 8–9

feedback design for treatment 8–9
first-drink criterion 152, 153
follow-up participation 73, *74*, 75
Aftercare arm 140–1
Form-90 drinking assessment instrument 34, 35, 152, 153
reliability/validity 188–9
FRAMES motivational enhancement therapy 46

gamma-glutamyl transpeptidase (GGTP) 32, 152, 153
gender 66
matching hypotheses 91
outcome prediction 6, 7
prognostic effect 142, 228
therapists 229
group therapy 49–50

homeopathy 3–4
hope 234

Important People and Activities interview 34
individual therapy 49
informants, collateral 41
inpatient treatment 18
instrument selection criteria 33–4
interpersonal dependency 98
Interpersonal Dependency Inventory, Assertion of Autonomy subscale 98
interpersonal interactions 12
interventions for alcoholism 3–4

ambulatory 81
intensity 13

language problems 72
latent growth analysis 108–9
liver function tests 39, 46, 152, 153

matching hypotheses 81–2, 84–5, *86–9*, 90–102
a priori 83, 84, 110–11
Aftercare arm 146
prognostic effects across time 116, *118–19*
Aftercare arm 135–49
clinical significance 146–7
testing 143, *144*, 145
alcohol dependence 96–7
alcohol involvement 85
anger 97
antisocial personality disorder 97–8
approval process 83–4
Bonferroni correction 84
causal chains 83, 213–14
choice criteria 83
cognitive impairment 85, 90
conceptual level 90–1
development 82–4
gender 91
interpersonal dependency 98
measurement of characteristics 33
motivation 92
primary 83, 84, 85, *86–7*, 90–6
prognostic effects across time 116, *118–19*
psychiatric severity 93
psychopathology 99
readiness to change 99–100
religiosity 100
secondary 83, 84, *88–9*, 96–102
prognostic effects across time 116, *118–19*
self-efficacy 100–1
social functioning 101–2
sociopathy 93–4, 97, 98
statistical procedures 82
supported 218–19
tests in Outpatient arm 117, *120–1*, 122, *123*, 124, *125*, 126
tiers 83
see also treatment matching
McAndrew Alcoholism Scale 46
meaning seeking 91–2, 231
hypothesis 100, 143
prognostic effect 215
motivation
alcohol dependence correlation 178

motivation (*cont.*)
  behavioral change 39, 45, 92
    intentional 177–9
    internal 23
  matching hypotheses 92
  predictor of outcome 116, 175, 181, 228
  prior AA attendance correlation 178
  time effect *120*, 122
  Working Alliance correlation 178
Motivational Enhancement Therapy
    (MET) 23, 41, 45–7, 169, *170*, 171
  AA attendance 192–5
    frequency 202
  alcohol dependence 96–7
  anger 97, *120*, 124, 212, 219, 231
  antisocial personality disorder *120*, 122
  behavioral change 92
  choice of therapy 224
  client satisfaction with treatment 176
  clinical deterioration 59
  compliance 54
    outcome association 78
  costs 59–61
  crisis strategies 58
  interpersonal dependency 98
  meaning seeking 143
  motivation time effect *120*, 122
  outcome 211
  psychiatric severity hypothesis 129
  psychopathology 99
  readiness to change 100, 145
  sessions 46
  social functioning 101
  sociopathy outcome 94
  support for drinking *120–1*, 122
    hypothesis 131
  therapeutic dimensions *56–7*
  therapists 46–7, 52, 171–2
  treatment effects 115, 219
  treatment manual 50
  treatment matching 223
  trends over time 139, *140*, *141*
  typology of alcoholism 95
motivational psychology 23
multi-level latent growth process 108–9
mutual-help groups 230

National Institute on Alcohol Abuse and
    Alcoholism (NIAAA; US) xiii, 13,
    238, 242
  alcoholism treatment expert panel
    17–18
  clinical trials 15
  funding 17–18
neuropsychological functioning 35
  test performance 46

order effects 39
outcome measures
  analyses 132
  composite 152, 153
  drinking behavior alternative measures
    154, *155–6*, 157, 163–4
  drinking frequency 138
  follow-up of clients 210
  latent growth analysis 108–9
  predictors 116–17
  proportional hazards analysis 154
  relapse rate 154, *155–6*
  secondary 158, *159*
    inter-relatedness 158–9
    multiple regression analysis 160, *162*
    post-treatment drinking relationship
      159–60, *161–2*, 163
  statistical analysis 107–12
  treatment effects 115–16
Outpatient arm
  AA attendance 190–2, 193, *194*, 195,
    217
    pro-drinking support networks 227
  AA utilization pattern 197–9
  abstinence 225
  alcohol and drug use 157
  ambulatory interventions 81
  causal chain analysis 128–31, 133
  client participation 25, *26*, 27
  client–treatment matching 212
  clinical deterioration 59
  clinical trial 20–1
  composite outcome measures 154, *155*,
    156, 157
  counseling 105
  deaths 59
  differences from Aftercare arm 225–7
  drinking reduction 131–2
  exclusion criteria 30
  exploratory analysis 126–8
  follow-up 25, 73, *74*, 75
    3-year 133
  inclusion criteria 29–30
  matching effects 148
  matching hypotheses tests 117, *120–1*,
    122, *123*, 124, *125*, 126
  outcome measures 107, 132
    primary 164
  participants 106–7
    enrollment 63, *64*, 65
    phase of life 164
    selection factors 164–5
  pro-drinking support networks 227
  prognostic effects 228
    across time 116–17
  recruitment 106–7, 226

research design 26
secondary outcome measures 158, *159*
self-efficacy 180
sites 217–18
statistical analysis 107–12
time to first drink 154, *156*
treatment
  choice 224–5
  effects 115–16
treatment manual 51
treatment outcomes 58, 218, 226
trends over time 113–15
Working Alliance Inventory 174, 175
outpatient treatment 18
clinical trial 20–1
intensive program use 226
use in USA 21, 226

Paragraph Completion Method 91
participants
after treatment 210
Aftercare arm 137–8
allocation procedure 67
collateral reports 75, *76*, 77
compliance 72
enrollment 63, *64*, 65–7
  alcohol problem severity 66
follow-up 73, *74*, 75
incentives 72
matching factors 6
motivation 230
orientation to research role 71
Outpatient arm 106–7
rewards 72
satisfaction with treatment 176–7
self-reports 75, *76*, 77
severity of disorders 209
treatment interaction 167–8, 233–4
working alliance 172, 173–5
see also client characteristics
Percent Days Abstinent (PDA) 32, 35, 107
AA attendance 200, 201
Aftercare arm 138, 139, *140*
exploratory analyses 126, 127–8
follow-up analysis 112, 140
secondary outcome correlation 160, *161*
self-efficacy 180
treatment effects 116
trends over time *113*, 114–15
performance indicator monitoring 19
pharmacotherapy 22–3
procedures, standardization 68
procedures manual 68
professional guidelines, matching treatment
  9
prognostic indicators 215, 228

prognostic variables 30–1
Project MATCH xiii–xvi
AA meeting attendance 227–8
abstinence 220
alcohol problem severity 66
assessment battery 34–5, *36–7*, 38
best practice 228–30
causal inferences 235
clients after treatment 210
clinical assessment 29–41
  instrument selection 33–4
clinical deterioration guidelines 58–9
collaborating facilities 239–40
collaborating investigators 239
committees 19
communication 20
consultants 239
cooperative agreement mechanism
  13–14
Coordinating Center 17, 18, 20
costs of therapies 59–61
credibility 208–9
Data Safety and Monitoring Board 240
deaths 59
effectiveness in community 226–7
exclusion criteria 29, 30, 66, 67
executing study xiv
Executive Committee 19
external validity 49–50, 79
follow-up participation 73, *74*, 75, 210
framework 16–17
funding xiv, 13–14, 17–18
genesis 3–14
inclusion criteria 29–30, 66, 67
initiation 15
internal validity 49–50, 79
interpretation of results xiv
methodology 235–6
mission-oriented approach 235–6
organizational structure 17–20
outcomes 210
  treatment differences 211
parallel studies 20–1
participant enrollment 63, *64*, 65–7
planning xiv
prognostic characteristics 228
project management 19
rationale 13–14
release of findings xiv
reliability assessment 69–70
research compliance 73, *74*, 75, *76*, 77
  correlates 77
research design 20–5, *26*, 27
  critical decisions 21–5
research personnel 240–2
sites 217–18

Project MATCH (*cont.*)
  Steering Committee 19, 20, 81, 82
    hypothesis adoption 83–4
  support service costs 60
  therapists 242–3
  therapy personnel 242
  therapy selection 42–50
  treatment
    choice 223–5
    delivery 208–9
    efficacy mechanisms 233
    implementation 50–5, *56–7*, 58
    matching 223
    measure choice 208
  treatment manuals 50–1
  working groups 19
  see also Aftercare arm; Clinical Research
    Units (CRUs); Outpatient arm
Project MATCH Research Group xiii,
    xiv, 17–19
  Leeds (UK) symposium xv
proportional hazards analysis 154
protocol implementation 20
psychiatric assessment timing 39
psychiatric disorders
  concurrent 8
  prognostic value 216
psychiatric severity 93
  change measures 153
  hypothesis 93
    causal chain analysis 129
    client–treatment matching 212
    clinical significance of matching 129
    outcome over time *120*, 122, *123*, 124,
      126
    treatment effectiveness 133–4
psychological functioning assessment 35–6
psychology, motivational 45
psychometric instruments, validated 31
psychopathology
  hypothesis 99
  treatment 93
Psychosocial Functioning Inventory
  Behavior subscale 101
  social role demands 153
psychosocial therapy 22, 166
psychotherapy 11
  technology model 233
  treatment outcomes 168
Purpose in Life (PIL) scale 92

questionnaires, test–retest reliability 70

readiness to change 99–100
  Aftercare arm 145
  measure 70, 92

motivational 35, 145, 175
  prognostic effect 215, 228
  predictor of outcome 116
  see also behavioral change
Recognition 100
recruitment strategies 63
regression testing 82
rehabilitation programs, residential 135
relapse
  outcome measures for rate 154, *155–6*
  process 100
  vulnerability and intentional behavioral
    change 177
relationally focused interventions 12
religiosity 100
  prognostic effect 142, 215
Religious Background and Beliefs scale
    70, 100
research activities, participation 71–3, *74*,
    75, *76*, 77–80
research compliance 73, *74*, 75, *76*, 77
  correlates 77
research protocol implementation 62,
    68–80
  participation in research activities 71–3,
    74, 75, *76*, 77–80
research site location 72
research staff
  compliance enhancement strategies
    71–3
  data processing/management 70–1
  measurement reliability 69–70
  supervision 68–9
  training 68–9

Seeking of Noetic Goals (SONG) scale 92
self-efficacy 35, 100
  Aftercare arm 143, *144*
  client–treatment matching 213
  intentional behavioral change 177, 180
  predictor of outcome 181
  prognostic effect 142, 215, 228
self-reports
  corroboration 34
  sensitivity 79
self-selection 8
Shipley Institute of Living Scale 31, 35
  Abstraction subscale 90
site effect covariates 110
sobriety, AA goal 185, 227
social functioning 101–2
  alcohol consumption relationship 160,
    162
  exploratory analysis 127–8
  outcome measures 124
Social Functioning Index 102

social instability 13
social learning theory 23, 43
social networks
  AA meeting attendance outcome 227
  prognostic effect 228, 231–2
  see also Support for Drinking hypothesis
social role demands 153
social support
  assessment 35
  perceived 70
sociopathy 93–4, 97, 98
  prognostic value 216
spirituality 35, 231
  prognostic effect 215
Stages of Change Readiness and Treatment
    Eagerness Scale (SOCRATES)
    100, 130
State–Trait Anger Inventory 97
statistical procedures 82
  Aftercare arm 138–9
  Bonferroni correction 83, 109, 143
  Outpatient arm 107–12
    covariates 109–10
    follow-up analysis, 3-year 112
    missing data 111–12
    a priori hypothesis tests 110–11
  stepped-care approaches 9
  Support for Drinking hypothesis 117,
    120–1, 122, 126
    AA attendance outcome 227
    causal chain analysis 130–1
    client–treatment matching 212
    clinical significance 130–1
    prognostic effect 228, 231–2
    social networks 130–1
  support services, costs 60
  Symbol–Digit Modalities Test 31, 35, 90

taking steps 100
Tape Rating Scale (TRS) 54
theoretically derived hypotheses 9, 10
therapeutic alliance 55, 58
therapeutic relationships, sociopathy 94
therapists 166, 171–3
  certification 53
  change process 234
  characteristics 172–3
  client interactions 168
  client outcomes 214
  Cognitive–Behavioral Therapy 45, 52
  costs 60
  crisis strategies 58
  deleterious effects 234–5
  gender 229
  Motivational Enhancement Therapy
    46–7, 52

personnel 242–3
recovering alcoholics 229
  role in recovery process 229
selection 51–2
skillfulness 55, 58
supervision 53, 167, 208–9
training 52–3, 167
traits 214
treatment
  outcomes 172–3
  variability 182
treatment manuals 50, 166–7
  Twelve Step Facilitation 49, 52
working alliance 172, 173–5
therapy selection 42–50
  cognitive–behavioral therapy 43–5
  criteria 42–3
time to first drinking event 152
Trail Making Test Part B 90
training seminars 68–9
treatment 169, *170*, 171
  access to 225
  attendance 178
  choice 223–5
  client interaction 167–8, 233–4
  clinical deterioration guidelines 58–9
  coerced referrals 65
  compliance 53–4
    enhancement strategies 71–3
  decisions 8
  delivery 167
  dimensions 169
  discriminability 54–5, *56–7*, 169, *170*,
    171
  effects across multiple dimensions of
    outcome 150–65
  efficacy mechanisms 233
  evaluation 151
  failure 5
  gender-specific 6, 7
  generic 6, 7
  intensity 164
  nonspecific components 55, 58
  patient interactions 233
  process assessment 38
  purifying 50
  random assignment 67
  research xv
  satisfaction of client 176–7
  sessions
    emergency 58
    monitored 53
    videotape rating 54
  standardization 229–30
  subsequent utilization 33
  success factors 225

treatment (*cont.*)
  triage 8
  unique components 55, 58
  universal elements 225
treatment manuals 50–1, 68, 208
  standardization 229–30
treatment matching 4–5, 223
  to clinical heterogeneity 3–14
  clinical significance 128–31
  disordinal 6–7
  hypothesis 5–6
  initiation of treatment 10
  measurement of variables 31, 33
  observed effect 13
  order effects in studies 39
  outcome 42
  previous studies 11–13
  rehabilitation intervention 11
  research 230–5, 236
  stages 10–11
  strategies 7
  theory 230–5
  during treatment process 10–11
  before treatment starts 10
  see also matching hypotheses
treatment outcomes 210
  AA attendance 91
  aftercare adjunct 21
  Aftercare arm 135–49
  assessment 25
  assessment battery effect 40
  client characteristics 215–16
  cognitive impairment 90
  compliance association 77–80
  composite measure 33
  covariate analysis 109–10
  decline in drinking 131–2
  defining 152
  deleterious effects 234–5
  drinking behavior alternative measures 154, *155–6*, 157, 163–4
  homogeneity 182
  matching 42
  measurement 31–2
    Type 1 error 32
  multidimensional view 151
  negative consequences of drinking 32
  predictors 6, *7*
    motivation 116, 175
  psychotherapy 168
  sociopathy 93–4
  statistical analysis 107–12
  therapist characteristics 172–3
  treatment differences 211
  treatment effects across multiple dimensions 150–65

trends over time 113–15, 139, *140*, *141*
unitary approach 151
variables 32–3, 70
see also outcome measures
triage 8
trust 234
Twelve Step Facilitation (TSF) 23, 47–9
  AA attendance 55, 169, 171, 187, 192–5
  client behavior 202
  enhancement 227–8
  frequency 202
  outcome 227–8
  abstinence 163, 220, 231
  emphasizing 146
  alcohol dependence 96, 97, 147
  anger *120*, 124
  antisocial personality disorder *120*, 122
  causal chain analysis 231
  choice of therapy 224–5
  client satisfaction with treatment 176
  clinical deterioration 59
  compliance 54
    outcome association 78
  continued involvement in activities 47
  costs 59–61
  crisis strategies 58
  drinking behavior alternative measures 163
  effectiveness 187
  follow-up 140
  gender 91
  interpersonal dependency 98
  meaning seeking 143
  objectives 48
  outcome 211
    variance prediction 217
  previous AA involvement 145
  psychiatric severity *123*, 124
    hypothesis 129
  psychopathology 99
  readiness to change 100
  religiosity 100
  sessions 48–9
  social functioning 101
  sociopathy outcome 94
  support for drinking *120–1*, 122
    hypothesis 131, 212
  techniques 169, *170*, 171
  therapeutic dimensions *56–7*
  therapists 49, 52, 171–3
  treatment effects 115, 218–19, 220
  treatment manual 50–1
  treatment matching 223
  trends over time 139, *140*, *141*
  typology of alcoholism 95

typology, outcome measures 124

University of Rhode Island Change
   Assessment instrument (URICA)
   31, 92
   readiness to change 99–100

verbal report corroboration 34

videotape rating 54, 209

women, representation in project 66
working alliance 172, 173–5
   motivation correlation 178
   prediction of drinking 181
Working Alliance Inventory 130, 174–5

Lightning Source UK Ltd.
Milton Keynes UK
06 October 2010

160841UK00001B/126/P